MW00580634

Gait Disorders in Childhood and Adolescence

Gait Disorders in Childhood and Adolescence

DAVID H. SUTHERLAND, M.D.

Professor of Surgery
Division of Orthopedics and Rehabilitation
University of California at San Diego
School of Medicine

Chief of Orthopedic Surgery
Director, Motion Analysis Laboratory
Children's Hospital and Health Center
San Diego, California

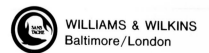

WILLIAMS & WILKINS
Baltimore/London

Editor: Barbara Tansill
Associate Editor: Victoria Vaughn
Copy Editor: William G. Vinck
Design: Joanne Janowiak
Illustration Planning: Wayne Hubbel
Production: Raymond E. Reter

Accurate indications, adverse reactions, and dosage schedules for drugs are provided in this book, but it is possible that they may change. The reader is urged to review the package information data of the manufacturers of the medications mentioned.

Made in the United States of America

Library of Congress Cataloging in Publication Data

Sutherland, David H.

Gait disorders in childhood and adolescence.

   Includes index.
   1. Musculoskeletal system—Diseases. 2. Musculoskeletal system—Abnormalities. 3. Neuromuscular diseases in children. 4. Pediatric orthopedia. I. Title. [DNLM: 1. Gait—In infancy and childhood. 2. Movement disorders—In infancy and childhood. 3. Gait—In adolescence. 4. Movement disorders—In adolescence. WE 103 S966g]
RD680.S9 1984   617'.398   83-10501
ISBN 0-683-08026-1

Composed and printed at the
Waverly Press, Inc.
Mt. Royal and Guilford Aves.
Baltimore, MD 21202, U.S.A.

TO MY WIFE, MILDRED

Preface

As an orthopaedic resident, I was fascinated by basic research on human gait conducted by the late Professor Verne Inman at University of California at San Francisco. The ability to measure movements, record electromyographic activity in muscles, and measure floor reaction forces seemed to offer powerful information which could be used clinically. Technical equipment and study methods at that time were not sophisticated enough for clinical application. However, the burgeoning of aerospace activities then taking place provided a base for conceiving and using new techniques in gait measurement. A large part of my professional life has been devoted to developing better methods of gait analysis and applying them to the study of patients with gait abnormalities. I am frequently asked, "How does gait analysis change your thinking about the treatment of patients?" The cases cited in this book are intended to convey the manner in which gait measurements have shaped my thinking and influenced the process of decision making with respect to my patients.

The study of gait disorders can be a source of continuous stimulation and challenge. Two levels of skill in disease pattern recognition can be attained. The first level of proficiency is the ability to identify common disease entities from visual recognition of disordered movement. An observer with this degree of skill can identify hip joint malfunction through observation of lateral shift of the trunk during single-limb support. This trained individual can also identify lordotic posture, posterior arm alignment, extended knee and equinus posturing of a patient in the late ambulatory stage of Duchenne muscular dystrophy. Skills at this level are common among experienced orthopaedic surgeons, pediatricians, neurologists, physiatrists, and physical therapists.

The second level of understanding gait disorders involves a thorough knowlege of force plate values, movement measurements, and electromyography. These measurements provide the foundation for kinematic and kinetic analysis of gait abnormalities. With this information, the observer can make objective comparisons before and after treatment. Biomedical engineers have contributed extensively to this second level of understanding. Collaboration between clinicians and biomedical engineers greatly benefits patients with gait disorders.

This book begins with definition of terms and a description of study methods. Normal gait is then described in sufficient detail to permit comparison of pathological gait patterns with gait in normal controls (subjects). Individual examples have been chosen to demonstrate each disease entity included. The cases are taken from the files in the Motion Analysis Laboratory at Children's Hospital in San Diego. Front and side view tracings of individual 16 mm movie frames supply the visual pattern of movement abnormalities. Graphs of joint rotations, linear measurements, dynamic electromyograms, and floor reaction measurements are the basis of biomechanical analysis.

In many instances case reports include studies before and after treatment to demonstrate that most children with gait abnormalities can profit from physical therapy, orthopaedic surgery, orthotic management, or a combination of these modalities. Visual recognition, biomechanical analysis, the process of treatment selection, and the results of treatment are presented in most of the cases cited.

Acknowledgments

Many of the basic concepts of clinical gait analysis presented in this volume originated when I was director of the Gait Analysis Laboratory at Shriners Hospital for Crippled Children in San Francisco (1956–1972). John L. Hagy was a key participant with me in working out the photographic measurement system. Raymon Linder, Richard Oyama, and Cecil Keller, employees of Lockheed Aircraft Corporation Missiles and Space Company, Sunnyvale, California, also made significant contributions. John L. Hagy, John R. Hawthorn, and Cecil Keller developed the piezoelectric force plate. Roger Mann, M.D., assisted with developing both the photographic measurement system and clinical force plate analysis. Frederick Bost, M.D., Edwin R. Schottstaedt, M.D., and Loren J. Larsen, M.D., chief surgeons at Shriners Hospital, San Francisco, made possible clinical applications of study methods by their encouragement and support. The national Shrine organization provided financial support through a special research grant.

The establishment of a motion analysis laboratory at Children's Hospital in San Diego evolved from the cooperative efforts of Children's Hospital and the University of California at San Diego. Wayne H. Akeson, M.D., Professor and Head of the Division of Orthopedics and Rehabilitation at the University, encouraged the project and offered guidance in designing research protocols. Mrs. Percy H. Johnston and P. H. "Duke" Johnston generously donated the funds to construct and equip the laboratory.

The National Institutes of Health provided grant support for the research study on the development of walking—Grant HDO 8520. A research grant from the Muscular Dystrophy Association of America supported studies of progressive alteration of gait in Duchenne muscular dystrophy.

Savio Woo, Ph.D., Richard Olshen, Ph.D., Dale Daniel, M.D., and Scott J. Mubarak, M.D., gave valuable assistance in studies of normal children, analysis of calcaneal limp, and Duchenne muscular dystrophy research. They are coauthors in publications on these subjects. Alan R. Hargens, Ph.D., and Lawrence L. Malcom, Ph.D., also contributed to the research projects.

Patient studies in this book are drawn from case records in the Motion Analysis Laboratory at Children's Hospital in San Diego. I am indebted to the numerous physicians who referred their patients for gait analysis and permitted additional studies to assess treatment outcome. They have contributed materially to this text by sharing their patients.

Motion Analysis Laboratory personnel at Children's Hospital, San Diego, deserve considerable credit. Lester B. Cooper, B.A., Project Engineer, assembled the electronic equipment, wrote the computer software for movement measurement, torque, and work output programs, and kept the studies moving. Marilynn P. Wyatt, M.A., R.P.T., research physical therapist, assisted in preparing research protocols, assessed subjects for muscle strength and contractures, conducted the studies, including insertion of internal electromyographic electrodes, and was coauthor in research publications. Research technicians Craig Breuninger, Patricia Dedrick, Susan Millard, Don Nothdurft, and Lesley Wise performed gait studies and reduced data. Edmund N. Biden, D.Phil., the present bioengineer, refined the measurement techniques and strengthened quality control in the laboratory. Secretarial assistance for the gait studies was provided by Sherill Marciano.

Patricia Dedrick did the illustrations. Her familiarity with the patients and measurement techniques was invaluable.

I wish to express my appreciation to Kaye Barlow who began preparing the manuscript and to Elizabeth Wright who edited and completed the major part of the work.

Final credit goes to the parents and children. Without their cooperation, this book would not have been possible

Contents

CHAPTER 1

Laboratory Methods and Terminology*

INTRODUCTION

There are many excellent techniques and methods for analyzing human walking. The methods described in this book are limited to those used in studying the subjects presented here. Both adults and children are seen in the Motion Analysis Laboratory, but the context of this book will relate to children.

Gait studies involving children should be performed by trained personnel who are relaxed and efficient. In this laboratory, a physician first examines the subject and selects the tests to be used and specific muscles to be studied. A research physical therapist examines the patient and records contractures, muscle strength, and passive range of motion. The therapist places the electrodes and supervises the subject during the test procedures. A research technician, under the supervision of a bioengineer, operates the equipment and subsequently reduces all data. The physician summarizes the findings and makes recommendations.

The laboratory is a comfortable setting, with wall graphics and toys designed to put children at ease and gain their confidence. The equipment, including cameras, force plate, electromyography equipment, and floodlights, is permanently mounted and ready for immediate operation. Attention can be directed to patients without time-consuming "setting-up" procedures. Parents are encouraged to remain throughout testing, although some parents choose to leave during insertion of electromyographic electrodes.

The process of data gathering and analysis used in the Motion Analysis Laboratory at San Diego Children's Hospital will be described. Material from a gait analysis conference at Long Beach, California, in 1979, provides information on the advantages, disadvantages, and costs of current methods available in this field (3).

TEST PROCEDURES

The subjects wear brief underclothing so that markings can be applied to help identify joint levels (Fig. 1.1). Test procedures are

---

* Portions of this chapter were taken from D. H. Sutherland et al.: *Journal of Bone & Joint Surgery*, 62A:336–353, 1980 (7).

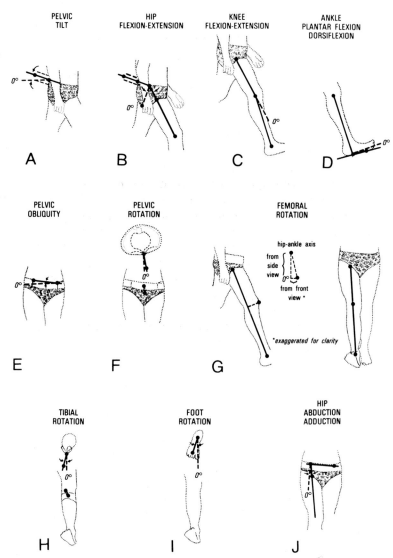

Figure 1.1.   Methods used to determine the various joint rotations. *Large dots* indicate actual measurement points and *broken lines* show the 0° reference for each angle. The drawings for femoral rotation show neutral rotation. Hence, the center of the front of the patella falls on the hip-ankle axis and no perpendicular line segment is visible in the front view (see text). (Reproduced with permission from D. H. Sutherland et al.: *Journal of Bone & Joint Surgery* 62A:336–353, 1980 (7).)

always performed with subjects barefoot, but when appropriate, additional studies are done with orthoses or special shoes. A sacral stick is attached to a thermoplastic base which is placed over the sacrum. A pelvic belt with a 5-mm wooden stick mounted perpendicularly in the center of the front piece is placed on the subject at the level of the hips. Tibial sticks are attached to thermoplastic bases molded to fit over the anterior aspect of the proximal end of the tibia. The walkway is at one end of a 21-m (70 ft) hallway with branching hallways extending from the site of the force plate to permit placement of the side viewing cameras (Fig. 1.2). A 2.7-m run-in allows the subject to attain normal walking speed before reaching the walkway. The area from which measurements are made is 3.4 m long. This length allows recordings of two to five strides, depending on the age and size of the subject. A run-out, more than 4 m long, assures that the subject slows down only after leaving the measured walkway area. A piezoelectric force plate 61 cm square is set in the floor 1.1 m from the beginning of the walkway. The force plate surface is made of plexiglass, 3.2 cm thick, which allows motion pictures to be made of the bottom of the foot using the pit camera.

The gait analysis laboratory includes three major subsystems: optical, electronic, and computer (7).

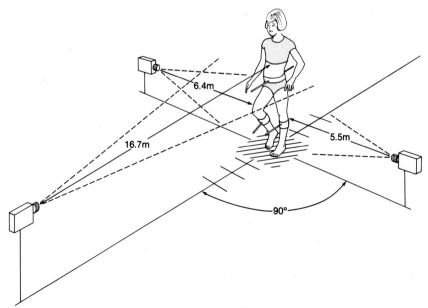

Figure 1.2. Arrangement of cameras and force plate in the gait laboratory (see text). (Reproduced with permission from D. H. Sutherland et al.: *Journal of Bone & Joint Surgery*, 62A:336–353, 1980 (7).)

OPTICAL SYSTEM

The motion-recording system includes four 16-mm motion picture cameras and a motion analyzer. The front camera is a Photosonics 1P recording camera with a 75-mm lens, which is placed 16.7 m from the center of the force plate and is centered on the longitudinal axis of the walkway. The left camera, also a Photosonics 1P, but with a 16-mm lens, is placed 5.5 m from the center of the force plate and is oriented perpendicular to the walkway. The right camera is a Hycam Model 40 high speed camera with zoom lens set at 18 mm. This camera is placed 6.4 m from the center of the force plate, perpendicular to the walkway (Fig. 1.2). The pit camera located beneath the force plate is a Bolex H16-RX 5 equipped with a 25-mm lens. To make a motion picture of the bottom of the foot during the stance phase of gait, this camera is aimed at a mirror that is placed at a 45° angle beneath the plate.

The front and side cameras are run at a speed of 50 frames per second, while the pit camera is run at 24 frames per second. The cameras run independently. A digital time display unit, which indicates seconds and tenths of seconds, is placed in the field of view of each camera so that time measurements can be taken from the film and used to verify camera speeds.

Processed film is displayed on a Vanguard motion analyzer which provides a rear-projected image of the subject on a viewing screen. The film is viewed frame by frame or may be advanced at up to 30 frames per second. A Science Accessories Graf-Pen sonic digitizer is used in conjunction with the motion analyzer to determine the x and y coordinates of the positions of the markers on the viewing screen (Fig. 1.3). The sonic digitizer is an acoustic coupler device, composed of a sound source, two microphones (one mounted along the top and the other along one side of the viewing screen), and electronic circuitry that measures the time taken for the sound to travel from the source to the microphones. To obtain the position of a marker on the screen, the observer places the sound source over a measurement position (such as the center of the knee) and activates the digitizer by pressing a button to begin the measurement cycle. In this cycle, the sound source emits a sound pulse and the time taken by the sound to travel from the source to each microphone is measured and is converted into units of distance in the x and y directions (Fig. 1.4). The coordinates of the point are recorded on a magnetic tape cassette automatically after each conversion. The observer then moves the sound source to the next point and begins another measurement cycle.

ELECTRONIC SYSTEM

The major elements of the electronic system are the force plate and the electromyographic system. The force plate is composed of seven piezoelectric load cells arranged to provide outputs produced by the

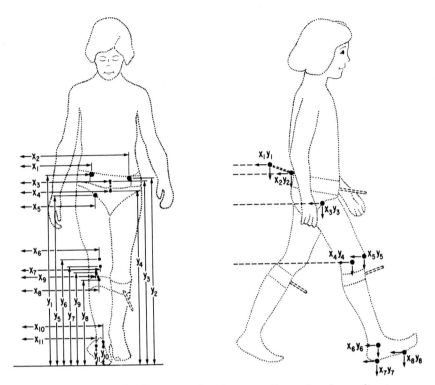

Figure 1.3. Front and side views showing two-dimensional coordinate map used when right gait cycle film data are read on the motion analyzer. *Subscripts* identify the order in which the data points are taken and later identified in computer calculations. The zero reference lines for the x and y coordinates are established by the Graf-Pen sonic digitizer. (Reproduced with permission from D. H. Sutherland et al.: *Journal of Bone & Joint Surgery,* 62A:336–353, 1980 (7).)

forces in three planes: vertical, fore-aft, and medial-lateral. The manner in which the output signals are recorded allows the computer to calculate the torque about a vertical axis going through the center of pressure as well as the vertical force, fore-aft shear, and medial-lateral shear (7).

The electromyographic system includes motion control MC-1 surface electrodes, a Tektronix oscilloscope, a Soltec oscillograph, and the Hycam camera previously described (7). The recording of surface muscle group activity is accomplished with surface electrodes, but deeper muscles such as the iliacus and the tibialis posterior are not accessible for surface recording. Furthermore, EMG potentials from individual muscles cannot be isolated with accuracy (2). For these reasons internal electrodes are mandatory when EMG information is sought for the planning of muscle releases or muscle transfers. Four

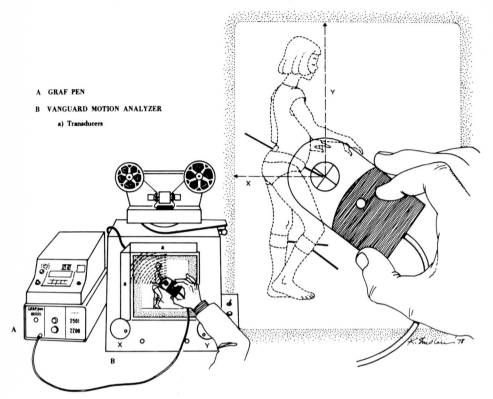

A GRAF PEN

B VANGUARD MOTION ANALYZER

   a) Transducers

Figure 1.4. Vanguard motion analyzer and Graf-Pen sonic digitizer used to determine the x and y coordinates of the markers shown on the viewing screen. (Reproduced with permission from D. H. Sutherland et al.: *Journal of Bone & Joint Surgery,* 62A:336–353, 1980 (7).)

muscles can be monitored at one time with our equipment. The electrodes are placed over the muscles, and the signal is displayed on both the oscilloscope and the oscillograph. As the subject walks along the walkway the electrical activity of the muscles is recorded on the oscillograph. In addition, a signal that indicates the time of heel-strike is produced by switches placed on each heel of the subject. The Hycam camera records the subject's movements through one lens and the muscle activity, which appears on the oscilloscope screen, through another lens. In this manner it is possible to correlate muscle activity with the subject's movement.

COMPUTER SYSTEM

A D.E.C. PDP 11/44 computer performs all calculations once the data are converted to digital form. The results of the calculations, which can be presented in either graphic (x-y plotter) or tabular (line printer) form, are stored for future analyses.

PARAMETERS MEASURED

The measurements of angular rotation are made throughout the left and right walking cycles of each subject. The following four measurements are made using only the views obtained with the side camera.

Pelvic Tilt

This measurement is made by means of the sacral stick. From the side view, the positions of the tip and of the base of the stick are measured. Neutral pelvic tilt (0°) is recorded when the stick position is parallel to the floor. Increased pelvic tilt occurs as the tip of the stick rises above the base of the stick (Fig. 1.1A), and decreased tilt is recorded when the tip moves in the opposite direction.

Hip Flexion-Extension

This measurement is the angle between the line segment formed by the line between the hip and knee center. If this angle is 90°, the hip flexion-extension angle is recorded as zero. An angle of more than 90° indicates hip flexion, while an angle of less than 90° represents hyperextension (Fig. 1.1B).

Knee Flexion-Extension

This is measured as the angle formed by the line segments between the hip and knee centers and between the knee and ankle centers. When the two line segments are in a straight line (Fig. 1.1C), 0° of flexion (full extension) occurs.

Ankle Plantar Flexion-Dorsiflexion

This angle is formed by the line segment between the knee and ankle centers and the line along the bottom of the foot. Neutral (0°) is the position when the two line segments form a 90° angle. Angles greater than 90° indicate plantar flexion; those less than 90°, dorsiflexion (Fig. 1.1D).

The remaining measurements are made on the film from the front view camera with the exception of femoral rotation, which requires use of both front and side views.

Pelvic Obliquity

This measurement uses the spots on the front of the pelvic belt. If the spots fall on a line parallel to the floor, the pelvic obliquity is 0°. If the marker on the right is higher than the one on the left, the pelvic obliquity is recorded as up for the right side or down for the left (Fig. 1.1E) and vice versa.

Pelvic Rotation

The stick projecting from the front of the pelvic belt is used for the measurement of pelvic rotation. If the tip and base of the stick are in line as seen from the front view, the rotation is recorded as 0°. Internal pelvic rotation for the right side and external rotation for the left side of the pelvis (Fig. 1.1F) occurs when the tip of the stick rotates to the right of center as seen from the front (to the subject's left) and vice versa.

Femoral Rotation

To make this measurement it is necessary to take readings from the front and side views at the same times during the cycle. From the side view, a line segment is defined which intersects the center of the front of the patella and is perpendicular to the line between the hip and ankle centers (Fig. 1.1G). From the corresponding front view, a second line segment is defined in similar fashion. This intersects the center of the front of the patella and is perpendicular to the line between the hip and ankle centers (Fig. 1.1G). These two line segments (front view and side view) are then used to determine the angle of rotation of the hip. Since these two line segments establish two sides of a right triangle (in a plane parallel to the floor), an angle of rotation can be calculated by trigonometry. In general, the angle of rotation is zero if the markers for the hip, center of the patella, and ankle are in a straight line as seen from the front. Internal rotation is measured if the patella is turned toward the midline of the body with respect to the hip-ankle line. External rotation is measured when the patella is turned in the opposite direction.

Tibial Rotation

The positions of the tip and base of the tibial stick are measured. If the tip and base are in line as seen from the front, the rotation is zero. Internal rotation is recorded when the tip of the stick rotates toward the midline of the body (Fig. 1.1H). External rotation is the reverse.

Foot Rotation

The measurement points for foot rotation are the center of the ankle and the marker placed between the second and third metatarsal heads. When these two points are in line as seen from the front view, the rotation is zero. When the front of the foot rotates toward the midline of the body, the rotation is said to be internal (Fig. 1.1I). When the foot rotates in the opposite direction, the rotation is external.

Hip Abduction-Adduction

This motion is measured in terms of the angle formed by the line segment between the marker spots on the pelvic belt and by the line segment between the hip and knee centers. If the resulting angle is 90°, the angle of hip abduction-adduction is zero. Angles of more than 90° are abduction, while those of less than 90° are adduction (Fig. 1.1J).

Hip Rotation

This measurement is the difference between pelvic rotation and femoral rotation.

Knee Rotation

This measurement is the difference between femoral rotation and tibial rotation.

In addition, the following data are determined: time of opposite toe-off (percent of walking cycle); time of opposite foot-strike (percent of walking cycle); duration of single-limb stance (percent of walking cycle); walking velocity (centimeters per second); cadence (steps per minute); step length (centimeters); stride length (centimeters); cycle time (seconds); and ratio of pelvic span to ankle spread (measured during the double-limb support phase).

DATA ANALYSIS

At least three passes down the walkway are observed on the motion analyzer. Each pass includes about three full walking cycles. The data from the measurements of the three passes are averaged, and the walking cycle that most closely approaches the average is selected for analysis. The measurements used to determine a representative cycle are: cadence, cycle time, step length, duration of single-limb stance (as percent of gait cycle), and the percent of the cycle at which toe-off, opposite toe-off, and opposite foot-strike occur.

The observer begins the reduction of the data by projecting the right side view film frame showing heel-strike on the motion analyzer. Eight points on the side view film frame are digitized (Figs. 1.3 and 1.4): the tip of the sacral stick, the base of the sacral stick, the center of the hip joint, the center of the knee joint, the patellar marker, the center of the ankle, the bottom of the foot beneath the heel, and the bottom of the foot near the fifth metatarsal head. The film is advanced two or three frames, as required, to give evenly spaced measurement increments throughout the cycle. (For example, if a walk cycle consists of 54 film frames, the film is read every third frame, giving 19 nearly equally spaced measurements.) The digitizing process is continued until the walk cycle is complete, and then the corresponding front view film frame showing heel-strike is projected on the motion analyzer and the 11 points on this view are digitized (Fig. 1.3): the right pelvic-belt spot, the left pelvic-belt spot, the base of the pelvic stick, the tip of the pelvic stick, the center of the hip joint, the center of the knee, the patellar marker, the base of the tibial stick, the tip of the tibial stick, the center of the ankle, and the marker between the second and third metatarsals on the dorsum of the foot. The film is then advanced and the readings are repeated on each view until the walking cycle is complete. When the digitizing for the right side view and front view films of the cycle is complete, the process is repeated for the left side view.

The cassette tape with the digitized information is transferred into the computer through another tape player and x-y coordinate data are used to calculate the angular rotations for the left and right walking cycles.

REPRODUCIBILITY

The same observer nearly always reproduces his or her measurements for each measured point to within 3°. Between observers there is seldom a difference for any measured point that is greater than 5°.

DEFINITIONS

The gait cycle is defined as the movements and events that occur between successive footsteps of the same foot. In normal subjects the gait cycle begins with heel-strike, continues through stance phase and swing phase, and ends with heel-strike of the same foot. In pathological gait the forefoot may make the initial floor contact to begin the gait cycle. Figure 1.5 illustrates a gait cycle of a 7-year-old normal subject (6). Stance phase ends with toe-off which initiates swing phase. Swing phase ends with foot-strike. Opposite toe-off and opposite foot-strike are the other significant gait events which create the separation of stance phase into periods of initial double support, single-limb stance, and second double support. Reversal of fore-aft shear provides one more separation of single-limb support into mid stance and terminal stance. It is not possible to make this last separation accurately without a force plate. Swing phase is separated into three periods: initial swing, mid swing, and terminal swing by two events. The first event is movement of the swinging ankle beyond the opposite standing tibia and the second event is vertical alignment of the swinging tibia. It is important for the reader to be familiar with these subdivisions of gait. In many pathological gait studies the abnormal movements can be found in specific periods. In the individual case studies, the periods will be named, but only the events will appear on the graphs. It is assumed that the reader will be able to identify the periods when provided with the time of occurrence of the event. In order to allow comparisons between subjects, all of the events, phases, and periods of the gait cycle are given in percentage of the total gait cycle. This conversion to percentage normalizes the individual studies.

Phasic muscle activity is the period during the walking cycle when there is electromyographic activity of a muscle (percentage of cycle).

Duration of single-limb stance is defined as the duration of single-limb support during the walking cycle (percentage of cycle).

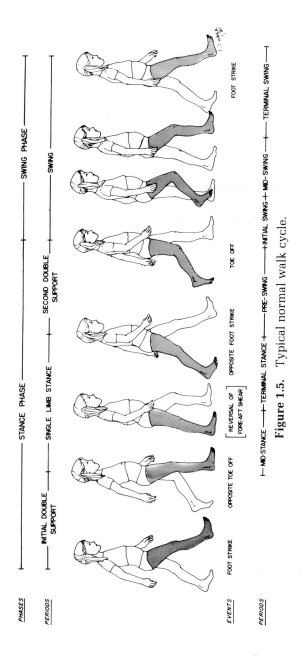

Figure 1.5. Typical normal walk cycle.

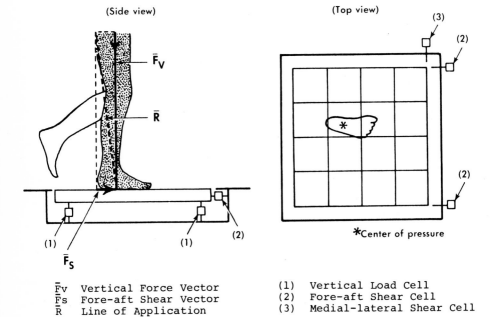

Fv   Vertical Force Vector
Fs   Fore-aft Shear Vector
R   Line of Application

(1)   Vertical Load Cell
(2)   Fore-aft Shear Cell
(3)   Medial-lateral Shear Cell

Figure 1.6. Determination of force vectors and center of pressure by force plate. (Reproduced with permission from D. H. Sutherland et al.: *Journal of Bone & Joint Surgery*, 62A:336–353, 1980 (7).)

Step length is the distance between the same point on each foot during double-limb support (in centimeters).

Stride length is defined as the distance traveled by the same point on the same foot during two successive steps. Therefore, each stride length is composed of one right and one left step length (in centimeters).

Cadence is the number of steps per minute.

Walking velocity is defined as the average distance traveled per second (in centimeters). It is determined by dividing stride length by cycle time.

Vertical force is the floor reaction force in the vertical direction as measured by the force plate.

Fore/aft shear is the floor reaction force acting horizontally in the line of progression.

Line of application of floor reaction force (R) is defined as the resultant of the vertical force vector $(\overline{F}_v)$ and of the fore-aft shear vector $(\overline{F}_s)$. The termination of the floor reaction force vector (R) is at the center of pressure (Fig. 1.6) (8).

Center of pressure is defined as the point of origin of the line of application of the floor reaction force calculated from force plate data.

Extrinsic joint torque is the torque produced by the forces of gravity and inertia and tends either to flex the joint if the line of application of the floor reaction force falls behind the joint, or extend the joint if the line of application of the floor reaction force falls in front of it (5, 8).

Intrinsic joint torque is the torque produced by the muscle forces tending to flex or extend the joint. For practical purposes with our present level of sophistication in measuring muscle forces, intrinsic joint torques are indeterminate. However, if movement of the joint is well controlled during stance phase, it can be assumed that there is some measure of equilibrium between extrinsic and intrinsic joint torques.

Work output is defined as the joules expended per kilogram of body weight per meter of distance walked. The work output is calculated from the force plate and film data by a modification of the method of Cavagna (1, 8).

References

1. Cavagna GA: Force platforms as ergometers. *J Appl Physiol* 39:174–179, 1975.
2. Perry J, Easterday KS, Antonelli DJ: Surface versus intramuscular electrodes for electromyography of superficial and deep muscles. *Phys Ther* 61:7–15, 1981.
3. Gait Analysis Conference. *Bull Prosthet Res* BPR 10–35: 279–320, 1981.
4. Sutherland DH, Cooper L: The pathomechanics of progressive crouch gait in spastic diplegia. *Orthop Clin North Am* 9:143–154, 1978.
5. Sutherland DH, Cooper L: Clinical use of force data. *Bull Prosthet Res* BPR 10–35: 312–315, 1981.
6. Sutherland DH, Cooper L: The events of gait. *Bull Prosthet Res* BPR 10–35: 281–282, 1981.
7. Sutherland DH, Olshen R, Cooper L, et al: The development of mature gait. *J Bone Joint Surg* 62A:336–353, 1980.
8. Sutherland DH, Cooper L, Daniel D: The role of the ankle plantar flexors in normal walking. *J Bone Joint Surg* 62A:354–363, 1980.

CHAPTER 2

Normal Walking

INTRODUCTION

Normal gait and the changes that occur with age must be clearly understood in order to appreciate the special features that characterize gait disorders in childhood and adolescence (10). For example, it is normal for a 1-year-old to walk with increased knee and ankle flexion, demonstrating flat-foot strike and absence of reciprocal swinging of the contralateral upper extremity with each footstep. However, this pattern in a 3-year-old child would suggest neuromuscular impairment.

The infant acquires the ability to sit at approximately 6 months, crawl at 9 months, walk with support at 11 months, and walk without support around 1 year of age. In the beginning phase of independent walking, the toddler steps with a wide base and hyperflexion of the hips and knees, holds the arms in abduction and the elbows in extension, and moves in a staccato manner. The width of the base diminishes gradually following the early exploratory phase of walking. Movements become smoother, reciprocal arm swing appears, step length and walking velocity increase, and an adult pattern of walking emerges (1, 2, 5, 8, 9).

Both learning and maturation of the central nervous system contribute to the development of mature gait. The course of maturation of the central nervous system progresses in a cephalocaudal manner (3, 4, 6, 7). From this, it may be deduced that motor control of the most distal segments of the lower extremity occurs after control has been established in the more proximal segments. This should bring about greater variation in the more distal movements than in the proximal movements—a phenomenon observed in a research study done in this laboratory (11).

The data base for age-related gait parameters and individual gait sketches which follow was derived from gait studies of 464 normal children between 1 and 7 years of age and 15 adults between 19 and 40 years of age. The study was supported by a National Institutes of Health grant and was carried out in the Motion Analysis Laboratory at San Diego Children's Hospital. Complete details of this study were presented in a previous publication (11). The 1-year-old girl shown in Figure 2.1A typifies the 51 children studied in this age group. This figure shows the tracing from individual movie frames at times of

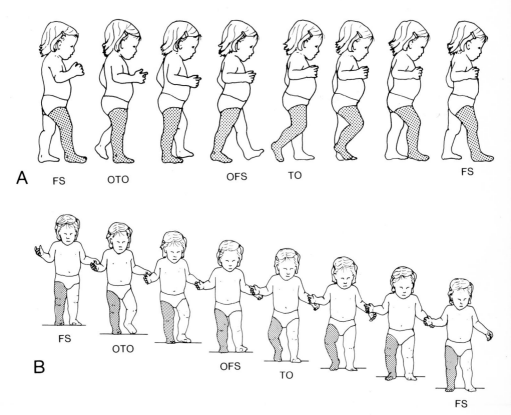

Figure 2.1. (*A*) Gait of 1-year-old girl. Tracings from individual movie frames throughout one full gait cycle. The individual frames coincide with significant gait events. Walk cycle begins with right foot-strike on the left and ends with foot-strike of the same foot on the right. (*B*) Frontal view (FS = foot-strike, OTO = opposite toe-off, OFS = opposite foot-strike, and TO = toe-off).

significant events throughout the gait cycle. The walk cycle begins with right foot-strike on the left and ends with right foot-strike on the right. Notice the flat foot-strike without the normal heel-strike of the mature walker. The elbows are maintained in flexion, and there is no evidence of reciprocal arm swing with contralateral footstep. The front view as shown in Figure 2.1*B* gives even greater evidence of gait immaturity. The arms are flexed and abducted. The base of support is widened, and the hips are externally rotated in swing phase. Additional linear measurements reveal a high cadence, low walking velocity, and short step length. A 1-year-old child does not have sufficient neuromuscular control to increase step length and an increase in cadence is the only mechanism for increasing velocity. Figure 2.2 shows the average joint rotations of 51 children in this age group. The

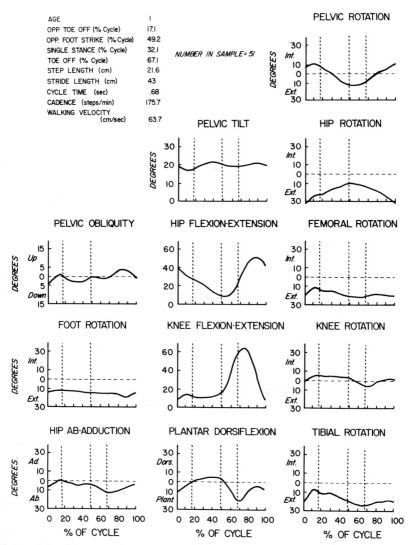

Figure 2.2. Joint rotations, 1-year-olds, right side. *Broken vertical lines (from left to right) indicate left toe-off, left foot-strike, and right toe-off.*

average time of significant events of gait, step length, stride length, cycle time, cadence, and walking velocity are also given.

The gait of 2-year-old children shows evidence of greater maturation as compared with that of the 1-year-olds. In the 2-year-olds, pelvic tilt and external rotation of the hip are diminished. The knee goes into greater flexion after foot-strike and then extends before toe-off in the so-called flexion wave. Heel-strike is present in a large number of the

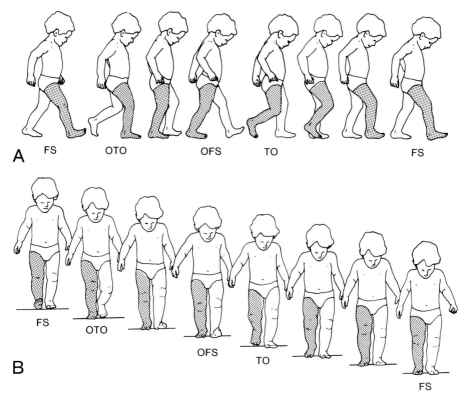

A   FS   OTO   OFS   TO   FS

B

FS   OTO   OFS   TO   FS

Figure 2.3. (A) Two-year-old normal male gait pattern demonstrates presence of heel-strike at the time of foot contact, reciprocal arm swing and greatly increased step length. (B) Frontal view (see Fig. 2.1 for abbreviations).

children, and the mild foot drop in swing phase noted in the 1-year-olds is no longer present. The 2-year-old male in Figure 2.3A demonstrates the gait pattern characteristic of this age group. This figure shows the presence of heel strike at the time of foot contact, reciprocal arm swing, and greatly increased step length. Figure 2.3B, frontal view, again demonstrates reciprocal arm swing and some decrease in the width between the ankles during double-limb support. Figure 2.4 shows the mean values for significant events of gait, the duration of single stance, and joint angles throughout the gait cycle for 45 normal subjects.

The average child displays an adult pattern of joint rotation by the age of 3 years. High cadence and low walking velocity are still present, and the duration of single-limb support is still below adult standards. With the exception of diminished stride length and abnormally high cadence, an adult pattern of walking has been achieved. The 3-year-old boy in Figure 2.5A shows a characteristic gait for this age group.

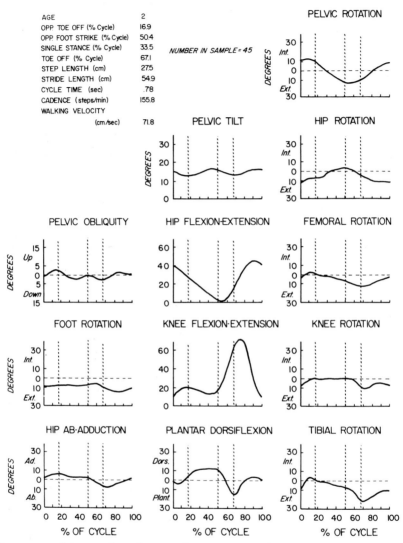

Figure 2.4. Mean values for significant events of gait and the duration of single stance and the joint angles throughout the gait cycle for 45 normal 2-year-olds.

This figure shows the vigorous gait, reciprocal arm swing, well-developed heel-strike, and smooth movements which differ only slightly from those of an adult. In Figure 2.5B, the base of support is narrow and rotation at the hip cannot be distinguished from that of an adult. In Figure 2.6, the average duration of single-limb stance, gait events, and joint angle rotations throughout the cycle are shown for 47 subjects in this age group.

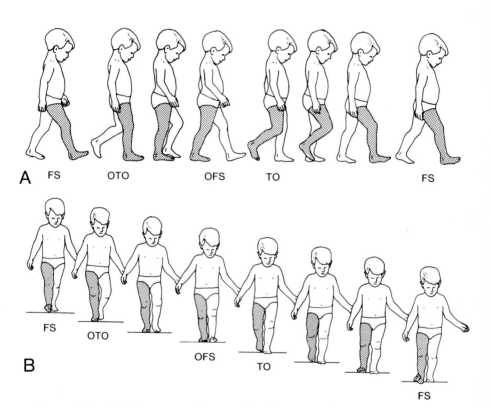

A   FS   OTO   OFS   TO   FS

B   FS   OTO   OFS   TO   FS

Figure 2.5. (A) Three-year-old normal male gait pattern shows vigorous gait, reciprocal arm swing, well-developed heel-strike and smooth movements which differ only slightly from an adult. (B) Frontal view (see Fig. 2.1 for abbeviations).

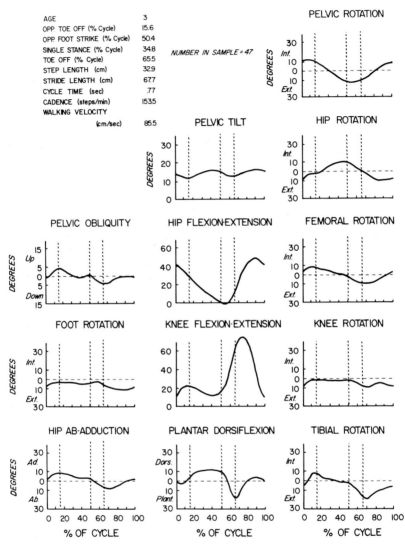

Figure 2.6. Mean duration of single-limb stance, events, and joint angle throughout the cycle are means for 47 normal 3-year-olds.

Except for increased stride length produced by increased limb length and accompanying reduction in cadence, the walk pattern of the 7-year-old child differs slightly from that of the 3-year-old's pattern. Figure 2.7A shows the tracings from movie frames of a 7-year-old girl. The movements of a mature walker are easily recognized and the front view (Fig. 2.7B) further confirms this. Figure 2.8 gives the mean values

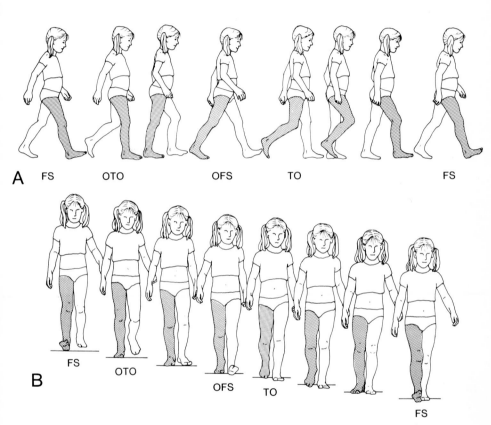

Figure 2.7. (*A*) Seven-year-old normal female gait pattern. (*B*) Frontal view (see Fig. 2.1 for abbreviations).

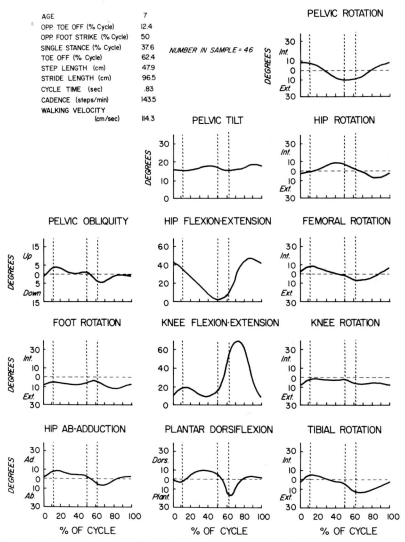

Figure 2.8. Mean values for gait events, during single stance, velocity, cadence, step length, and joint angles for 46 normal 7-year-old subjects.

for gait events during single stance, velocity, cadence, step length, and joint angles for 46 normal subjects.

It is clear by this time that joint angle normal controls need not be prepared for each year of growth after 7 years. To complete the picture, similar measurements of 15 normal adults are included. Figure 2.9, *A* and *B*, shows individual tracings from movie frames of a normal adult woman, age 25. Mean values for the 15 adults are shown in Figure 2.10.

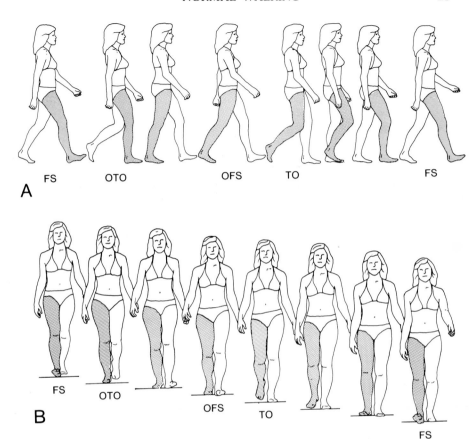

Figure 2.9. *(A-) Normal adult gait pattern.* (B) Frontal view (see Fig. 2.1 for abbreviations).

MUSCLE PHASIC ACTIVITY

The "muscle firing pattern" is called muscle phasic activity. Each muscle has a repeating, predictable, "on-off" time which is linked to the function it performs. The term "swing phase" or "stance phase activity" is not precise, since many muscles extend activity partially from one phase into another phase. On-off time is given in percentage of gait cycle, so that the exact events in movements occurring during the same time period can be correlated. The usefulness of correlating movements with muscle contraction time is shown by describing the function of the ankle plantar flexors as determined by simultaneous movement measurement, force plate analysis, and electromyography. The gastrocnemius and soleus contract from approximately 12% of the gait cycle to 50% when weight is transferred to the opposite limb. During this period of time, the ankle first continues to dorsiflex in spite of the lengthening reaction (eccentric) of the triceps surae, slows,

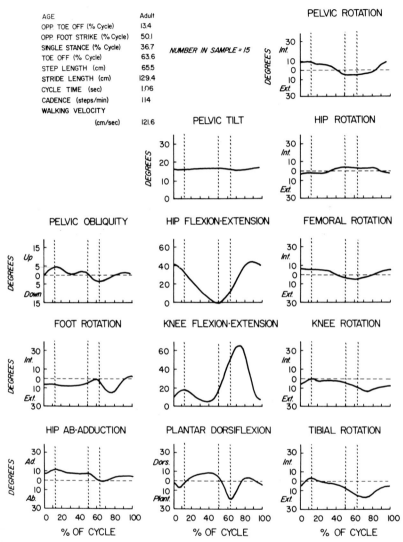

Figure 2.10.   Mean values for 15 adults.

stops, and then reverses, reducing the dorsiflexion. Muscle action ceases with transfer of weight to the opposite limb. With respect to the ankle joint, the muscle action decelerates and then accelerates (12). It is important to know when a muscle fires, but even more essential to know what happens during muscle action. Conclusions can then be drawn about the effect of muscle action upon movement. If a movement occurs while the muscle acts against the motion, the effect of the muscle action is deceleration (eccentric reaction). If the ends of the muscle come closer together through joint rotation in the direction of the muscle action, the muscle contributes to the movement (concentric reaction).

The force plate is a valuable tool which permits measurement of the line of application of floor reaction force, and (with movement measurement) its distance from the joint center. When this line falls behind the joint, flexion must be resisted if joint stability is to be maintained, and the muscles on the opposite side of the joint must react. In this laboratory, understanding the function of lower extremity muscles in walking has been illuminated by data which measure the line of application of floor reaction force. The lower extremity muscles oppose applied loads, and the on-off times of these muscles can be predicted by examining the time of transition of the force line from flexion to extension or from extension to flexion. The force plate has now become a powerful implement in linking the action of muscles with kinetic forces.

There are no extensive studies of muscle phasic activity in children utilizing internal electrodes. It would be difficult to obtain the cooperation of small children in the tedious task of multiple fine-wire electrode insertions. The Motion Analysis Laboratory has chosen to establish normal phasic activity of muscle groups by using surface electrodes. For ages 1 through 7 (10 age groups, including 1½, 2½, and 3½-year-olds), the mean muscle phasic activity is shown for the seven muscles or muscle groups (11). These will be the normal standards against which children from 1 to 7 years of age will be compared. Established adult electromyographic standards will be used for children above the age of 7 or where single muscles or muscles not included are studied (Fig. 2.11).

The muscle phasic activity of children is similar to adults. However, in the two youngest age groups studied in our laboratory (1 year, 1½ years), EMG phasic activity began prematurely in swing phase in the vastus medialis and gastrocnemius/soleus, and there was stance phase prolongation in the gluteus maximus, vastus medialis, lateral and medial hamstrings, gastrocnemius/soleus, and tibialis anterior (11). These variations in muscle phasic activity, which are accompanied by the gait abnormalities found in the earliest stages of walking, are likely caused by lack of proper motor control which is dependent upon myelinization.

THE FIVE IMPORTANT DETERMINANTS OF MATURE GAIT

Our studies have shown that joint angles measured throughout the gait cycle are weak determinants of mature gait. The sagittal plane joint angles are very similar to normal adults by age 2 ½ years. There are five strong determinants: duration of single-limb stance, walking velocity, cadence, step length, and the ratio of pelvic span to ankle

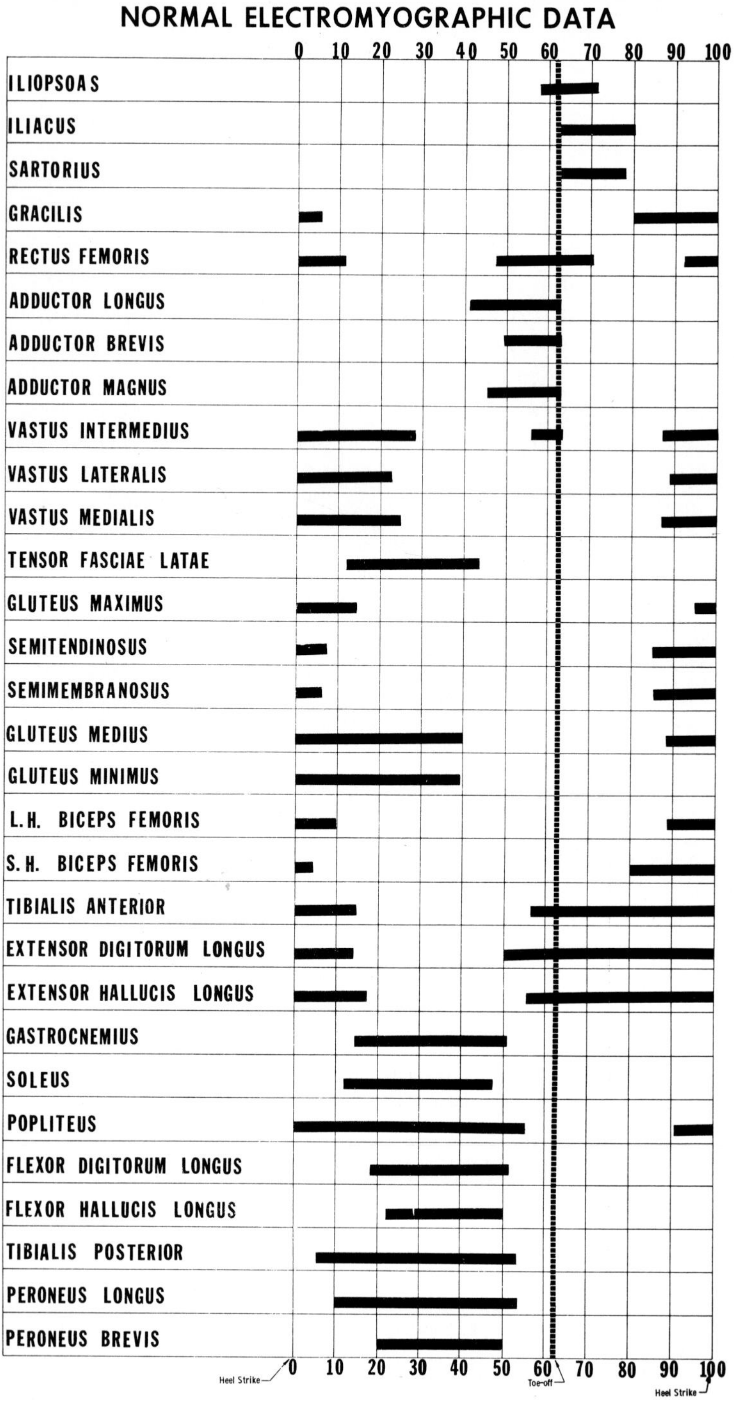

NORMAL ELECTROMYOGRAPHIC DATA

Figure 2.11. Adult muscle phasic activity chart—Shriner's Hospital, San Francisco.

26

spread. The normal values of these determinants in children between 1 and 7 years of age are found in a previous publication (11). Increases occur with progressive age in the duration of single-limb stance, walking velocity, step length, and the ratio of pelvic span to ankle spread. However, cadence drops with progressive age. The greatest changes occur during the first 4 years of life.

DISCUSSION

Gait maturation occurs rapidly in children. Heel-strike, knee flexion wave, reciprocal arm swing, and an adult pattern of joint angles throughout the walking cycle are all acquired before the development of mature cadence, step length, walking velocity, duration of single-limb stance, and ratio of pelvic span to ankle spread (1, 2, 11). Maturity can be judged by these five latter determinants. Muscle phasic alterations in the early walkers are likely due to faulty motor control caused by lack of complete myelinization.

Our understanding of the normal sequence of events plus the existence of accurate measurements of gait parameters for each age group are prerequisites for the pathological gait studies. In each instance comparisons will be made with age-related normal subjects.

References

1. Burnett CN, Johnson EW: Development of gait in childhood. Part I. Dev Med Child Neurol 13:196–206, 1971.
2. Burnett CN, Johnson EW: Development of gait in childhood. Part II. Dev Med Child Neurol 13:207–215, 1971.
3. Conel JL The Postnatal Development of the Human Cerebral Cortex. Cambridge, Harvard University Press, Vol IV, 1951.
4. Conel JL: The Postnatal Development of the Human Cerebral Cortex. Cambridge, Harvard University Press, Vol V, 1955.
5. Gesell A: The First Five Years of Life. New York, Harper & Row, 1940.
6. Longwerthy OR: Development of behavior patterns and myelinization of the nervous system in the human fetus and infant. In Contributions to Embryology, vol. XXIC, No. 139. Publication No. 443, pp. 1–57. Washington, Carnegie Institute, 1933.
7. Peiper A: In Nagler B., Nagler H. (eds): Cerebral Function in Infancy and Childhood (translated from the third edition). New York, Consultants Bureau, 1963.
8. Sheridan MDS: The Developmental Progress of Infants and Young Children, Ministry of Health Report No. 102. London, H.M. Stationery Office, 1961.
9. Statham L, Murray MP: Early walking patterns of normal children. Clin Orthop 79:8–24, 1971.
10. Sutherland D: The value of normative data in gait analysis, NIH Gait Research Workshop. DHEW Publication No. NIH 78-119. Childrens Hospital, San Diego, Calif, March 1977.
11. Sutherland DH, Olshen R, Cooper L, et al: The development of mature gait. J Bone Joint Surg 62A:236–253, 1980.
12. Sutherland DH, Cooper L, Daniel D: The role of the ankle plantar flexors in normal walking. J Bone Joint Surg 62A:254–263, 1980.

CHAPTER 3

Rotational Deformities

INTRODUCTION

Intoeing is the most common problem seen by the orthopaedist in the pediatric age group (15). Parental anxiety on this subject usually centers about the belief that difficulties will arise in adult life from lack of attention to rotational abnormalities of childhood. Orthopaedic surgeons and pediatricians realize that few adults have significant rotational abnormalities without an associated orthopaedic defect, and the conclusion is that spontaneous resolution usually occurs. While some articles in the orthopaedic literature suggest that long-term degenerative changes are based on rotational abnormalities (6, 10), proof of this has not been demonstrated. Parents sometimes associate clumsiness with internal rotation, but again there is no evidence that the two are directly related.

The question of physical performance and excessive idiopathic femoral anteversion was studied by Staheli and others (14). Nine adults with clinical evidence of excessive idiopathic femoral anteversion and 10 age- and sex-matched controls were studied. All subjects underwent a 3-week conditioning program, after which performance was evaluated by the following tests: 1) running performance—50- and 440-yard dash, shuttle, circle, and zig-zag run; 2) static balance; 3) speed of limb movement; and 4) explosive strength by standing long jump. Another group of 249 high school students, ages 14–18, was studied to compare running speed. Excessive idiopathic femoral anteversion was assessed by measuring hip rotation. Fifteen patients with the greatest difference between external and internal rotation were compared with the remaining group. The findings of this study indicated that running skills in the adolescent and adult are not adversely affected by moderate increase in femoral anteversion. In both studies there was no relationship between excessive anteversion and physical performance.

The ranks of professional athletes include individuals with increased internal rotation. There is no apparent difference between their performance and other players who are closer to the norm of rotation alignment.

Although most rotational abnormalities are benign in nature, careful musculoskeletal examination is mandatory. Serious orthopaedic problems such as hip subluxation or cerebral palsy may coexist with toe-in gait. After excluding more serious disease, the orthopaedist should establish the anatomic level and record any abnormal alignment. Femoral antetorsion, internal tibial torsion, and metatarsus varus are the three conditions which commonly produce intoeing (15). Theories explaining their incidence are: 1) intrauterine molding, 2) heredity, and 3) environmental factors such as sleeping and sitting patterns which impede the normal resolution of internal rotation (15, 19).

METATARSUS VARUS

Metatarsus varus is a common kind of birth deformation, milder in type but similar in origin to clubfoot and congenital muscular torticollis (9, 12). The lateral border of the foot is convex and increased separation of the great and second toes is often noted. Supination of the forefoot may also appear. In contrast with congenital clubfoot, the heel is never in varus and there is no fixed equinus. Foot deformity is flexible in milder cases, and stretching is enough to overcome the problem. Other cases require casting for correction. It is advantageous to complete casting before walking begins.

TIBIAL TORSION

Tibial torsion can be assessed by palpating the medial and lateral malleoli at the ankle, with the child sitting and the knee flexed to 90°. The transmalleolar axis obtained in this manner is compared with the axis of rotation of the knee joint. More accurate measurement can be made by using the Staheli method (7, 13). Tibial torsion averages 5° of external torsion during the first year, 10° during mid-childhood, and 14° in older children and adults (4, 13). Internal tibial torsion under 18 months of age seldom requires treatment. In a child over 18 months of age and under 3 years, the use of a splint with the feet set in external rotation may be helpful for increased internal tibial torsion. The splint modifies sleeping postures which delay the normal process of spontaneous correction (6, 19).

Internal Tibial Torsion

Patient M.G. was referred to a pediatric orthopaedic surgeon at the age of 19 months because of left intoeing. He was the product of a full-term pregnancy, with labor induced because of decreased amniotic fluid and decreased contractions. Birthweight was 8 lb and 4 oz. Independent walking began at 12 months of age. The parents complained that the child was tripping over the turned-in left foot.

Torsional profile modified from Staheli (15):

	Right	Left
Hip internal rotation	40	40
Hip external rotation	80	80
Thigh-foot axis	+15°	−10°
Foot	N	N

Tibial torsion measured by Staheli's method was +5 on the right and +7.5 on the left. Normal values of tibial torsion as measured in this laboratory for 1½-year-old children are: right-external, +4.7; left-external, +6.6. The discrepancy between tibial torsion measured by the thigh-foot axis and Staheli's method can best be explained by the influence of subtalar movement on foot alignment. The ankle joints and the heel must be held in neutral position, or significant errors will occur in thigh-foot axis measurement due to improper alignment of the subtalar joint.

Tracings of film from the left side camera showed increased elbow flexion, flat foot strike, and equinus in swing phase (Fig. 3.1A). Tracings of film from the front camera showed wide base of support, abduction of arms and bilateral intoeing (Fig. 3.1B).

Walking velocity was normal at 76 cm per second. Cadence was 148 steps per minute compared to the average for age of 177 steps. Stride length was 54 cm (average for age, 50 cm) (Fig. 3.1C).

Joint angle rotations in the left lower extremity differed from the normal for age in transverse plane rotations (Fig. 3.1C). External rotation of the pelvis and femur and internal rotation of the tibia and foot were noted.

Joint angle rotations of the right lower extremity (not shown) included abnormalities of transverse plane movement with internal rotation of the pelvis, external rotation of the femur, and internal rotation of the tibia and foot. The measured right foot progression angle (foot rotation) showed only slightly less internal rotation than the left.

This gait study highlights the difficulties in correct assessment of internal tibial torsion. Patient M.G. was diagnosed as having internal tibial torsion and is now being treated with a Denis-Browne bar. Although the left foot turns in and there is left internal tibial torsion by thigh-foot axis measurement, more accurate measurement of tibial torsion by the Staheli method did not confirm abnormal alignment.

Perhaps this case should have been excluded, since tibial alignment by Staheli's method was normal for age. However, the case was reported because it emphasizes the difficulty in evaluating tibial torsion accurately. It is probable that the child would do well without treatment.

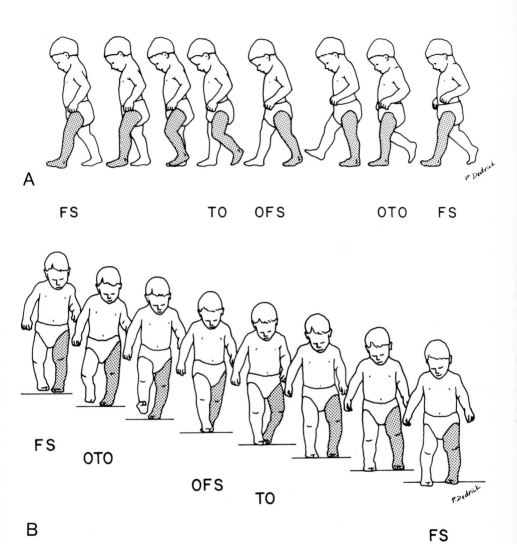

Figure 3.1. (A and B) Patient M.G., age 19 months: internal tibial torsion. Tracings of film from left side (A) and front (B) camera. (FS = foot-strike, TO = toe-off, OFS = opposite foot-strike, and OTO = opposite toe-off.)

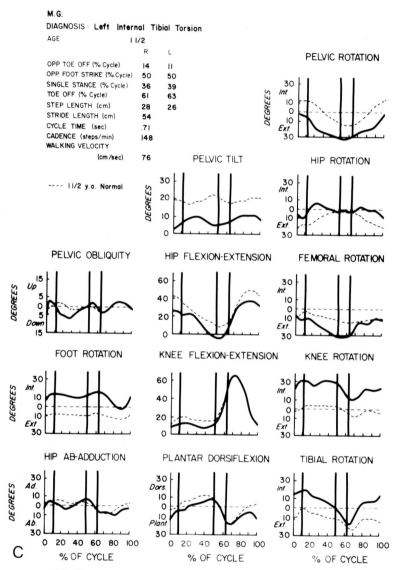

Figure 3.1. (C) Patient M.G. Linear measurements and joint angle rotations, left lower extremity. Values for 1½-year-old normal subject (*dotted line*) are shown for comparison.

FEMORAL ANTEVERSION

Abnormalities in development cannot be defined without precise information about normal development. Mean femoral anteversion which measures 40° at birth drops to 30° by the time a child is 2 years of age, 25° by 8 years, and 12° in adult life (5). The clinical test used most frequently to assess anteversion is comparison of external and internal rotation hip motion ranges with the subject in prone position (1). This test is inaccurate for a child under 2 years of age, because internal rotation of the hip is limited by factors extrinsic to the femur (11). The diagnosis of femoral antetorsion (exaggerated femoral anteversion) usually applies only to patients over three years of age. Accurate measurement of femoral anteversion requires radiographic assessment (2, 3, 8, 17, 18). For a child over 3 years of age, increased anteversion is more likely to cause intoeing than metatarsus varus or internal tibial torsion. There is no effective nonsurgical method of correcting femoral antetorsion, but few children with idiopathic femoral antetorsion require operative treatment (16). Spontaneous correction will take place even beyond 8 years of age, and consequently surgery should be the last resort. The complication rate for surgical derotation in 78 patients who underwent bilateral derotational osteotomy of the femur for medial femoral torsion was 15% (16). More compelling than the complication rate is the absence of proof that function is impaired and the lack of evidence of long-term degenerative changes in the hip or knee (16).

Patient G.G., a 5½-year-old child, was referred for pediatric and orthopaedic evaluation because of toe-in gait, learning difficulty, and bed-wetting. Prenatal and perinatal history was normal with the exception of some turning in of the foot noted soon after birth. At approximately 2 months of age, the child was placed in a Denis-Browne splint at night, and this treatment continued through the first year of life and part of the second. The parents felt that this improved but did not eliminate the toe-in tendency. Developmental milestones were normal. Walking began at 1 year.

Concern about the child's toe-in tendency, his immaturity, stuttering, and delay in toilet training prompted additional studies. Urological consultation yielded no findings to explain inconstant daytime incontinence and regular bed-wetting at night.

Torsional profile:

	Right	Left
Hip internal rotation	80	80
Hip external rotation	25	25
Thigh-foot angle	+7	+5
Foot	N	N

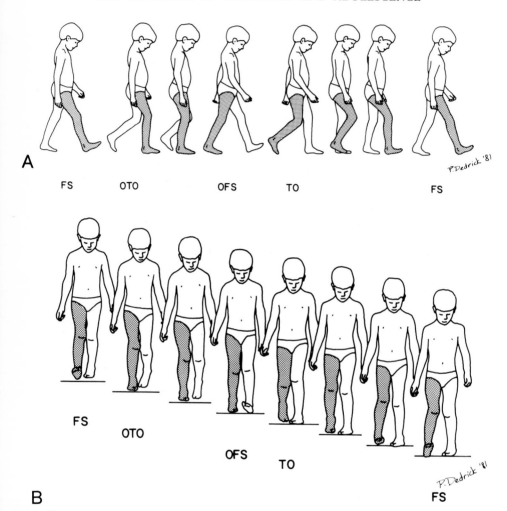

Figure 3.2. (A and B) Patient G.G., age 5½ years: idiopathic femoral antetorsion. Tracings of right (A) and front (B) camera film. (See Fig. 3.1 for abbreviations.)

Femoral anteversion measured by fluoroscopic method (18) was: right, 47°; left, 48°. These measurements indicated a 20° increase over the average value for this age.

Tracings of right camera film were not remarkable (Fig. 3.2A). Tracings of film from the front camera (Fig. 3.2B) showed bilateral intoeing from the hips. Linear measurements (Fig. 3.2C) differed only slightly from the 6-year-old normal values. The joint angles of the right lower extremity were compared with those of 6-year-old normal children. Internal hip rotation increased in stance phase. The foot

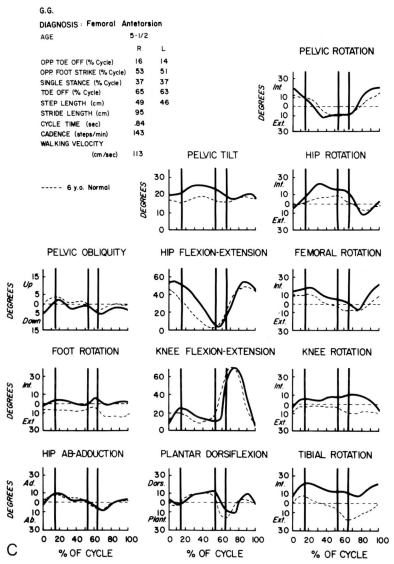

Figure 3.2. (C) Patient G.G. Linear measurements and joint angle rotations.

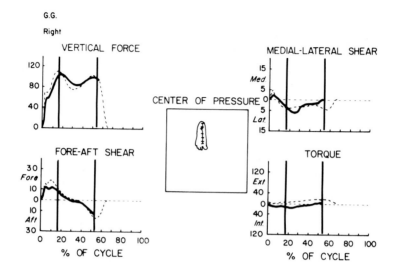

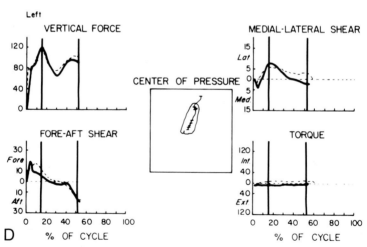

Figure 3.2.   (*D*) Patient G.G. Force plate measurement with normal for age comparison.

rotation angle was 0°, compared with the normal of approximately 8° of external rotation.

Force measurements did not differ significantly from normal values for age (Fig. 3.2*D*).

To summarize the gait findings, this child with measured anteversion (right, 47°, and left, 48°—a 20° increase over the average for age) walked with thighs internally rotated during stance phase, but with feet in neutral alignment (mild relative intoeing). The parents were advised that moderate idiopathic femoral antetorsion does not constitute a health hazard, function should not be affected, and no orthopaedic treatment was needed.

References

1. Crane L: Femoral torsion and its relation to toeing in and toeing out. *J Bone Joint Surg* 41A:421, 1959.
2. Dunlap K, Shands AR, Hollister LC, et al: A new method for determination of torsion of the femur. *J Bone Joint Surg* 35A:298–311, 1953.
3. Dunn DM: Anteversion of the neck of the femur: a method of measurement. *J Bone Joint Surg* 34B:181–186, 1952.
4. Engel GM, Staheli LT: The natural history of torsion and other factors influencing gait in childhood. *Clin Orthop* 99:12–17, 1974.
5. Fabry G, MacEwen GD, Shands AR: Torsion of the femur—a follow-up study in normal and abnormal conditions. *J Bone Joint Surg* 55A:1726–1738, 1973.
6. Knight RA: Developmental deformities of the lower extremities. *J Bone Joint Surg* 36A:521–527, 1954.
7. Le Damanay P: La torsion du tibia normale pathologique, experimentale. *J Anat Physiol* 45:598, 1909.
8. Magilligan DJ: Calculation of the angle of anteversion by means of horizontal lateral roentgenography. *J Bone Joint Surg* 38A:1231–1246, 1956.
9. McCormick DW, Blount WF: Metatarsus adductovarus. *JAMA* 141:449–453, 1949.
10. McSweeny A: A study of femoral torsion in children. *J Bone Joint Surg* 53B:90–95, 1971.
11. Pitkow RV: External rotation contractures of the extended hip. *Clin Orthop* 110:139, 1975.
12. Ponseti IB, Becker JR: Congenital metatarsus adductus: the results of treatment. *J Bone Joint Surg* 48A:702–711, 1966.
13. Staheli LT, Engel GM: Tibial torsion: a method of assessment and a survey of normal children. *Clin Orthop* 86:183–196, 1972.
14. Staheli LT, Lippert F, Denotter P: Femoral anteversion and physical performance in adolescent and adult life. *Clin Orthop* 129:213–216, 1977.
15. Staheli LT: Torsional deformity. *Pediatr Clin North Am* 24:799–811, 1977.
16. Staheli LT, Clawson DK, Hubbard DD: Medial femoral torsion: an experience with operative treatment. *Clin Orthop* 146:222–225, 1980.
17. Stewart SF, Karshner RG: Congenital dislocation of the hip: a method of determining the degree of antetorsion of the femoral neck. *AJR* 15:258–260, 1926.
18. Sutherland DH: A rational approach to proximal femoral osteotomy in children. *Proceedings, Leroy C. Abbott Orthopaedic Society, San Francisco* 6:60–68, 1975.
19. Thelander HE, Fitzhugh ML: Posture habits in infancy affecting foot and leg alignment. *J Pediatr* 21:306–314, 1942.

CHAPTER 4

Physiologic Genu Varum and Blount's Disease

INTRODUCTION

It is now common knowledge that bowlegs in infancy and early childhood are a normal part of development (7, 12–14). Salenius and Vankka (12) measured the tibial femoral angle of 979 patients from the Pediatric Clinic at the University of Helsinki and 300 patients from the Orthopedic Hospital of the Invalid Foundation in Helsinki. Many examinations were repeated on the same children, with a total of 1480 examinations. The mean tibial femoral angle at birth was 17° varus (Fig. 4.1). The mean time of transition from varus to valgus was 22 months. The mean time of maximal valgus angle was 3 years of age. After peak valgus, progressive reduction occurred, then leveling off at approximately 6½ years of age. Consequently, bowlegs in children under 2 years of age should not cause undue concern.

The usual pattern of spontaneous correction does not always apply, however. Some children progress from physiologic genu varum to tibia vara, or Blount's disease (2–5, 10). For reasons yet unknown, the normal process of conversion from varus to valgus fails and progressive dysplasia of the proximal tibia develops. If unchecked, this dysplasia leads to early growth arrest of the medial portion of the proximal tibial epiphyseal plate. The progressive stages of Blount's disease, as described by Langenskiold (10) are shown in Figure 4.2. It is theorized that progression from normal physiologic genu varum to Blount's disease is caused by exaggerated compression forces acting on the medial epiphyseal plate. An altered threshold of response to compression forces is an alternate but less attractive theory. Genetic factors must also be considered, since the condition is commonly found in the West Indies and Africa (1, 2, 6). Other factors may be early walking and obesity. Whatever the cause, there is agreement that osteotomy restores normal growth if the procedure is done in the early stages (3, 4, 10). Early bracing may also be effective in reversing progressive changes (3, 4, 9). The normal rebound from varus to valgus may be explained by Hueter-Volkmann's law (8). Compression of the medial epiphyseal plate during weight bearing stimulates growth, while unloading of the lateral portion of the epiphyseal plate inhibits growth. Failure of normal conversion from physiologic genu varum to genu valgum may be explained by excessive compression of the medial

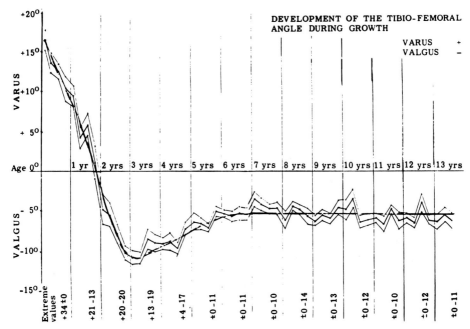

Figure 4.1.   The tibial femoral angle from birth to 13 years. (Reproduced with permission from P. Salenius and E. Vankka: *Journal of Bone & Joint Surgery,* 57A:259–261, 1975 (12).)

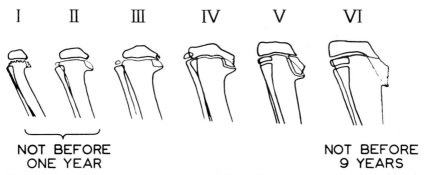

Figure 4.2.   The progressive stages of Blount's disease. (Reproduced with permission from A. Langenskiold and E. B. Riska: *Journal of Bone & Joint Surgery,* 46A:1405–1420, 1964 (10).)

epiphyseal plate which inhibits medial growth and produces varus alignment of the proximal tibia.

What constitutes excessive pressure and how can it be measured? How can early Blount's disease be distinguished from physiologic genu varum? There are no adequate answers to these questions, but gait studies with determinations of knee joint contact forces may provide answers in the future. Longitudinal studies of this kind are in process in the Motion Analysis Laboratory at Children's Hospital in San Diego, California. Most of the children in this study have converted spontaneously from genu varum to genu valgum without treatment. However, the condition of several children has worsened. Specific gait parameters are being examined to identify those changes in gait which herald the onset of Blount's disease. Just as hip dysplasia is reversible when normal hip joint contact force is restored, knee dysplasia growth can also be corrected by the same process. A thorough understanding of both normal growth and the pathomechanics of destructive forces acting through the knee joint will, in the future, allow early therapy in selected patients and prevent unnecessary treatment for the great majority of bowlegged children who will correct spontaneously.

The practitioner can detect rickets by history, clinical findings and x-rays, but the dilemma is how to distinguish between physiologic genu varum and early Blount's disease. The cases that follow will not suffice to answer this question, but the examples given may be helpful. One subject had physiologic genu varum which resolved spontaneously and another progressed from physiologic genu varum to Blount's disease.

PHYSIOLOGIC GENU VARUM

Patient D.F. was referred for gait analysis at 22 months of age because of a history of increasing bowlegs. His parents noted the exaggerated bowleg tendency at age 15 months. The subject first walked at 10 months and the condition was untreated. His vitamin intake was adequate in infancy and x-rays of the knees at 2 years disclosed no evidence of rickets. Examination revealed a healthy-looking 22-month-old boy with bowlegs. The intercondylar distance measured 6 cm with the patient supine. The transmalleolar axes as measured by the Staheli method were 0/0 (15).

A gait analysis was done and, after review of the results, observation was recommended with periodic additional gait studies. The five studies done showed the stages of gradual improvement. The initial and final studies were selected to demonstrate the spontaneous resolution of physiologic genu varum.

Figure 4.3A illustrates characteristic medial beaking of the femur and tibia seen in physiologic genu varum. Figure 4.3B shows film tracings in side view at 22 months of age. Signs of immaturity in walking were: 1) poorly developed reciprocal leg and arm swing, 2) increased hip and knee flexion at foot-strike, and 3) short step length. These were not gait abnormalities associated with physiologic genu varum, but simply evidence of incomplete maturation of gait (16). The

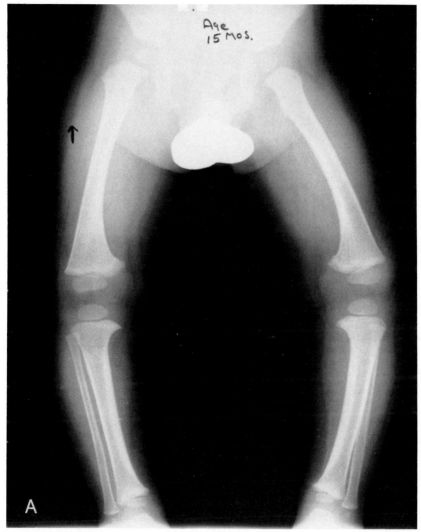

Figure 4.3. (*A*) Patient D.F., characteristic x-ray findings in physiologic genu varum at 15 months.

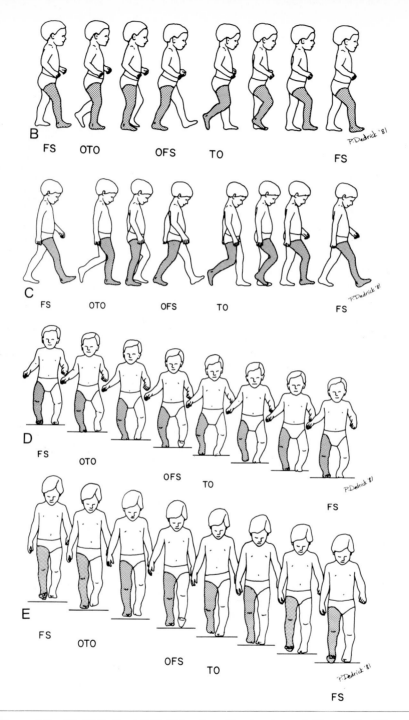

Figure 4.3. (*B–E*) Patient D.F. Side view film tracings at 22 months (*B*) and at 4 years (*C*). Frontal view tracings at 22 months (*D*) and at 4 years (*E*). Full spontaneous resolution of physiologic genu varum. Correction occurred without treatment. (FS = foot-strike, OTO = opposite toe-off, OFS = opposite foot-strike and TO = toe-off.)

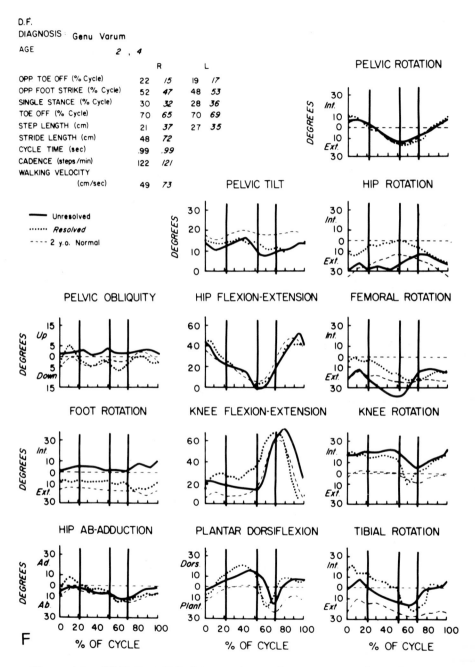

Figure 4.3. (F) Patient D.F. Joint angle rotations at 22 months and 4 years, shown together with average joint angle rotations of 2-year-old normal subjects.

side view of D.F. in Figure 4.3C at 4 years of age demonstrated a well-developed reciprocal arm and leg swing, overall increase in body height, and concomitant step length. Figure 4.3D (front view) at age 22 months shows bowleg alignment without varus thrust in single-limb support. Full resolution of the bowleg alignment appears in Figure 4.3E (age 4 years).

The joint angle rotations for this subject at 22 months and 4 years are shown, together with the average joint angle rotations of 2-year-old normal subjects (Fig. 4.3F). The cadence and walking velocity were lower than average at both ages, but probably exemplify the lack of achieving "free speed cadence," rather than reflecting impairment in walking. (Some children are self-conscious and occasional allowance must be made for failure to achieve "free speed cadence.") Patient D.F.'s joint angle rotations at 22 months of age are reasonably comparable to normal values in the 2-year-old (Fig. 4.3F). At 4 years, D.F.'s hip rotation curve demonstrated less external rotation of the hip in stance phase and slight external rotation of the foot in stance phase, replacing the earlier pattern of slight external rotation.

In summary, the findings in D.F. at 2 years of age deviated only slightly from the norm, even though his leg alignment was genu varum. External rotation of the hip and internal rotation of the knee were slightly increased in single-stance phase. All movements were normal by 4 years of age.

INFANTILE TYPE OF BLOUNT'S DISEASE

Patient J.M. was referred for orthopaedic evaluation at 2 years of age because of severe bowlegs. His early developmental history was normal, except that he walked at 10 months of age and bowlegs were observed at 12 months of age. By the time the patient was 2 years old, his parents were convinced that the bowleg tendency was getting worse. Examination revealed moderate genu varum. The transmalleolar axes as measured by the Staheli method were −3.75/−7.5 (internal tibial torsion) (15). X-rays revealed metaphyseal beaking and thickening of the medial cortices of the tibiae (Fig. 4.4A). The child walked with a rolling gait, with lateral thrust of the knees during weight bearing. A gait study was done, but no treatment was undertaken. A month later, the child returned and the bowleg condition was worse. A Denis-Browne bar was prescribed, and the parents were instructed to apply the bar at night. The child was reexamined in 2 months. The gait had not improved and the child continued to walk with a rolling gait and obvious lateral thrust of each knee during single-limb support. X-rays revealed an increase in dysplasia of the proximal tibiae, now consistent with Blount's disease, Stage II (Fig. 4.4B).

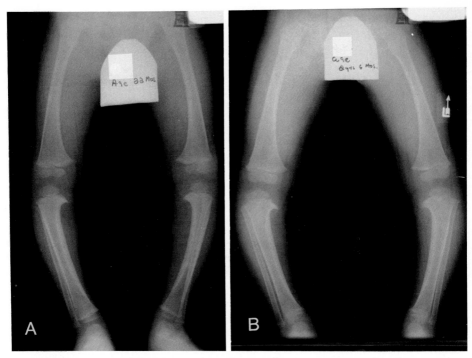

Figure 4.4. (*A* and *B*) Patient J.M.: Blount's disease. (*A*) At 22 months, x-ray shows Blount's disease, Stage I. (*B*) At 2 years and 6 months, x-ray shows Blount's disease, Stage II.

The gait study of this child at age 2 years and 7 months has been selected to represent the typical gait pattern of a child with the infantile type of Blount's disease. The lateral view does not reveal significant gait deviations (Fig. 4.4*C*), but the frontal view demonstrates significant gait abnormalities (Fig. 4.4*D*). There is an apparent increase in the genu varum alignment with limb loading. The femoral tibial angle is increased at opposite toe-off (OTO), as compared with foot-strike (FS). Increased lateral movement of the upper trunk and arm is particularly noticeable during single-limb support on the left. This lateral movement of the upper trunk and arm over the weight-bearing lower extremity moves the force line closer to the knee joint center, thus reducing the medial compressive force on the knee. This is a compensatory movement.

The sagittal plane joint angle rotations are normal for age (Fig. 4.4*E*). Marked deviations from normal are observed in the frontal plane movement of hip abduction-adduction which shows exaggerated abduction throughout the gait cycle. There is extreme external rotation

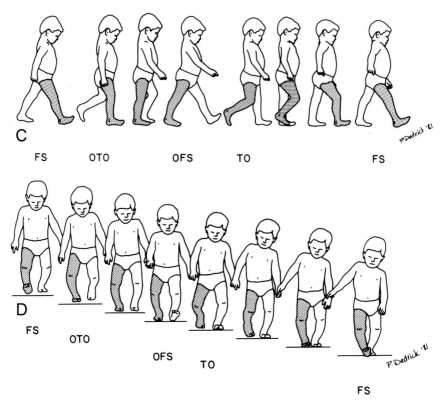

Figure 4.4.   (C and D) Patient J.M. at 2 years and 7 months. Film tracings from front side (C) and front (D) camera. (See Fig. 4.3 for abbreviations.)

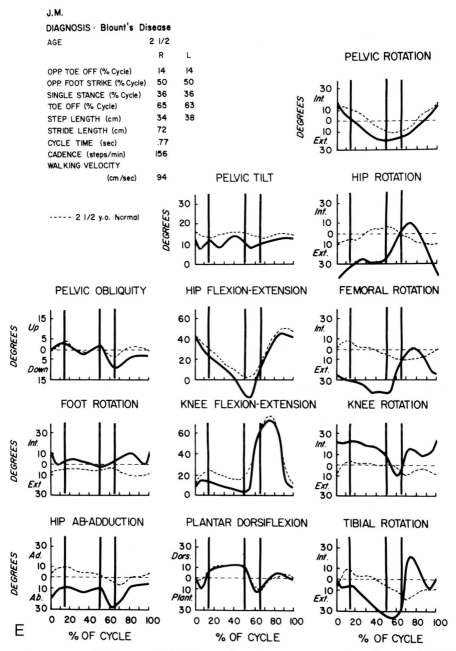

Figure 4.4. (E) Patient J.M. Joint angle rotations at 2 years and 7 months, comparison with mean of normal subjects as the same age.

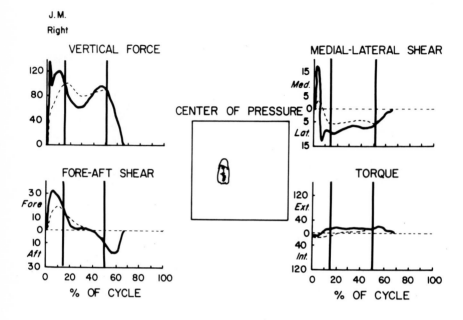

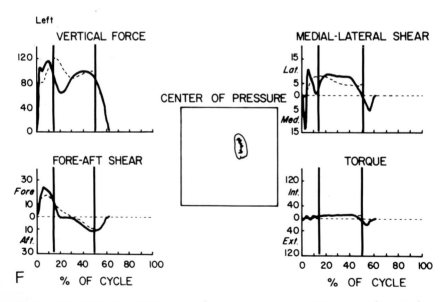

Figure 4.4.   (F) Patient J.M. Force plate measurements at 2 years and 7 months. *Dotted lines* represent mean values for normal subjects at 2 years and 6 months.

of the femur in stance phase, with marked external rotation of the hip joint through initial double and single limb support. During the same time period, internal rotation of the knee joint is increased.

Abnormalities in the force plate measurements appear in Figure 4.4F). Excessive vertical force and medial shear are noted in the right lower extremity, but increased medial shear alone is observed in the left lower extremity during the loading phase.

Following the second gait study, treatment was initiated, consisting of single upright long-leg braces without knee joints worn throughout each day, with continuation of the Denis-Browne bar at night. Under this regime, correction of genu varum is occurring, and osteotomy of the tibiae will be performed only if correction by bracing is delayed or incomplete.

SUMMARY

Infantile Blount's disease is a progressive disorder of growth of the proximal tibia produced by abnormally high compression forces acting across the medial portion of the knee joint in otherwise normal subjects. It must be differentiated from rickets and bone dysplasias of specific etiology, and seems to develop in children who show some exaggeration of physiologic genu varum. Movement abnormalities include: 1) excessive external rotation of the femur and hip joint, 2) excessive internal rotation of the knee joint, and 3) a peculiar lateral thrusting movement of the knee during single-limb support. Compensatory movement of the trunk and upper arms accompanies lateral thrusting of the knees. The purpose of these compensatory movements may be to bring the force line closer to the knee joint center and reduce the lateral movement of the knee. The majority of children with physiologic genu varum recover without treatment. Those children who need treatment are often overweight, beyond the age of normal conversion from varus to valgus, and show excessive external rotation of the hip, internal rotation of the knee, and lateral thrusting of the knee during single-limb support. Future studies will measure the extrinsic torques acting upon the knee joint in three planes of movement and the medial knee joint contact forces. These measurements will then provide a more scientific basis for prediction of growth dysplasia and selection of children who must be treated if progressive Blount's disease is to be prevented.

References

1. Bateson EM: Non-rachitic bow leg and knock-knee deformities in young Jamaican children. Br J Radiol 39:92–101, 1966.
2. Bateson EM: The relationship between Blount's disease and bow legs. Br J Radiol 41:107–114, 1968.

3. Blount WP: Tibia vara. *J Bone Joint Surg* 19:1–29, 1937.
4. Blount WP: Tibia vara: osteochondrosis deformans tibiae. *Current Pract Orthop Surg* 3:141–156, 1966.
5. Erlacher P: Deformierende Prozesse der 'Epiphysengegend bei Kind. *Arch Orthop Unfallchir* 20:81–96, 1922.
6. Golding JSR, McNeil-Smith JDG: Observations on the etiology of tibia vara. *J Bone Joint Surg* 45B:320–325, 1963.
7. Hansson LI, Zayer M: Physiological genu varum. *Acta Orthop Scand* 46:221–229, 1975.
8. Hueter C: Anatomische Studien an den Extremitatengelenken Neugeborener und Erwachsener. *Arch Pathol Anat* 25:572–599, 1962.
9. Kessel L: Annotations on the etiology and treatment of tibia vara. *J Bone Joint Surg* 52B:93–99, 1970.
10. Langenskiold A, Riska EB: Tibia vara (osteochondrosis deformans tibiae). *J Bone Joint Surg* 46A:1405–1420, 1964.
11. Pauwels F: Funktionelle Anpassung des Knochens durch Langenwachstum. *Dtsch Orthop Ges* 45:34–56, 1957.
12. Salenius P, Vankka, E: The development of the tibial-femoral angle in children. *J Bone Joint Surg* 57A:259–261, 1975.
13. Sherman M: Physiologic bowing of the legs. *South Med J* 53:830–836, 1960.
14. Shopfner CE, Coin CG: Genu varus and valgus in children. *Radiology* 92:723–732, 1969.
15. Staheli LT, Engel GM: Tibial torsion. *Clin Orthop* 86:183–186, 1976.
16. Sutherland DH, Olshen R, Cooper L, et al: The development of mature gait. *J Bone Joint Surg* 62A:336–353, 1980.

CHAPTER 5

Occult Limps

INTRODUCTION

What is a limp and how is it recognized? Many types of disease and injuries can produce limps and because the resulting abnormal movement is in the noninvolved limb, each limp becomes a challenge to the observer to localize the problem and identify the disease or injury. The opposite swinging limb is placed on the floor prematurely as a means of restricting the time of single-limb support. The painful or weak limb must be supported by the opposite limb which shares the load.

In visual gait analysis, the shortened opposite step and premature foot-strike of the opposite limb are telltale clues to pain or paralysis in the weight-bearing limb. Most limps are unilateral and produce asymmetry of stepping. Symmetrical bilateral limps are more difficult to recognize. The time of single-limb support and length of opposite step are the specific gait parameters most indicative of limping. These measurements must be made for both lower limbs to provide the proper basis for comparison. There should be a reduction in ipsilateral single-limb support and contralateral step length, as well as reduction of velocity and cadence in most instances. A reduction also occurs in the initial loading portion of the vertical force curve on the painful or weak limb in many cases. This usually takes the form of reduction in the magnitude and diminished slope of the first peak of the vertical force curve.

It is important to recognize that paralysis can also produce limps. Accordingly, proper muscle testing is an essential ingredient in successful diagnosis. In one type of paralytic gait—the calcaneal limp—the second peak of the vertical force curve is reduced because of insufficient muscle strength to permit transfer of weight to the forward portion of the foot during single-limb support. This subject will be discussed later, since the primary emphasis in this chapter is on limps produced by pain.

The following case reports illustrate a few common causes of occult limps, with the focus on specific gait parameters observed in the chosen examples.

DISCITIS

Patient R.M., a 2½-year-old boy, was admitted to Children's Hospital, San Diego, with a 3-week history of limp, irritability and anorexia.

Several days prior to admission, he had been crawling, although from time to time he resumed limited walking.

When the patient was placed in the left side-lying position with the right knee flexed, pain was produced by extension of the right hip (positive psoas test). A mild limp was observed in level walking, but a more obvious abnormality of movement occurred when he attempted to retrieve an object from the floor (Fig. 5.1A–C). During this maneuver, he maintained his spine in extension and approached the object by

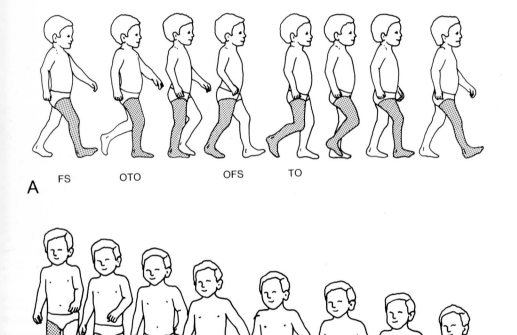

Figure 5.1. (A and B) Patient R.M.: discitis. Right angle gait cycle, side (A) and frontal (B) views. No gross abnormalities of movement are observed. (FS = foot-strike, OTO = opposite toe-off, OFS = opposite foot-strike, and TO = toe-off.)

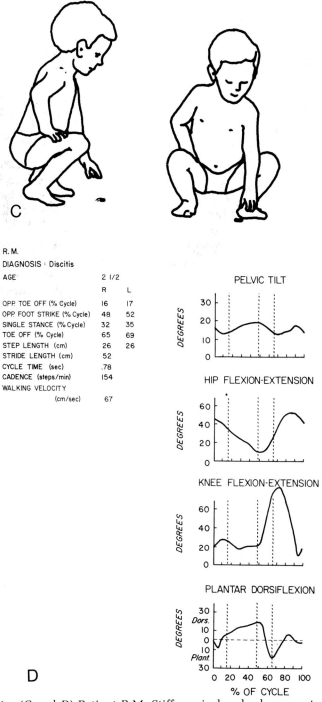

R. M.

DIAGNOSIS : Discitis

	R	L
AGE	2 1/2	
OPP. TOE OFF (% Cycle)	16	17
OPP. FOOT STRIKE (% Cycle)	48	52
SINGLE STANCE (% Cycle)	32	35
TOE OFF (% Cycle)	65	69
STEP LENGTH (cm)	26	26
STRIDE LENGTH (cm)	52	
CYCLE TIME (sec)	.78	
CADENCE (steps/min)	154	
WALKING VELOCITY (cm/sec)	67	

PELVIC TILT

HIP FLEXION-EXTENSION

KNEE FLEXION-EXTENSION

PLANTAR DORSIFLEXION

Figure 5.1. (C and D) Patient R.M. Stiffness in low back was noted during the act of squatting (C) to pick up an object from the floor. (D) Joint angle curves of right lower extremity during one walk cycle. The joint angles do not differ significantly from normal control values at age 2 (see Fig. 2.1).

flexing his knees and hips. Straight-leg raising on the right produced some pain at 70°, while there was no similar evidence of pain on the opposite side. The lack of flexion in the lower spine provided the clue to localizing the site of pathology.

Laboratory studies revealed WBC of 9.0/thousand; differential: neutrophils 43, lymphocytes 44, monocytes 5, eosinophils 8. The sedimentation rate was 50 mm per hour. A technetium-99m diphosphonate bone scan demonstrated increased activity over the lateral borders of the third and fourth lumbar vertebra. X-ray of the lumbar spine revealed disc space narrowing between L-3 and L-4.

Although this child was able to walk, many children with discitis stop walking because of pain before the diagnosis is made (4, 7). Cadence was normal for age, but walking velocity was reduced—67 cm as compared with an average of 81 cm (Fig. 5.1D). Stride length was reduced (52 cm as compared with an average of 62 cm). There was increased flexion of the right knee at foot-strike, but deviation was within normal variation. The joint angle rotation for ankle motion did not differ significantly from the average (Fig. 5.1D). The overall gait impression was that the child walked a little slowly because of back pain, but the clue to the cause was not revealed in the graphs of joint angle rotations.

FOREIGN BODY IN KNEE

Patient C.M., a 10-year-old boy, was admitted to Children's Hospital for removal of the head of a needle which had broken off in the posterior lateral aspect of the left knee joint. Previous attempts to remove the imbedded fragment at another hospital were unsuccessful. On admission, the child complained of mild pain and swelling of the knee.

Examination revealed tenderness over the lateral condyle of the left femur, a mild extension lag of the knee, and minimal quadriceps atrophy. X-rays showed a 3-mm lucent area containing the broken needle fragment in the lateral condyle of the left femur close to the joint surface. Gait analysis was performed before surgical removal of the foreign body. Following the surgery, the limp disappeared, with resolution of the symptoms.

The history of an unexplained limp accompanied by some tenderness about the knee should alert the examining physician to include the possibility of an imbedded foreign body in the differential diagnosis (1). This type of injury is not uncommon, and x-ray gives the diagnosis if the foreign body is metallic. In many instances, the parents are quite unaware of the mechanism of injury until an x-ray is obtained.

Asymmetry in stepping can be appreciated by comparison of the tracings taken at foot-strike (FS) and opposite foot-strike (OFS) (Fig.

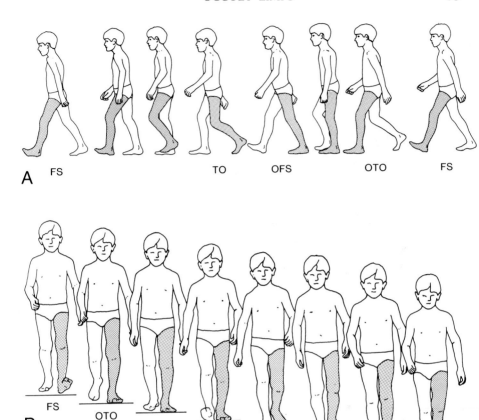

Figure 5.2. (A and B) Patient C.M.: foreign body in knee. Left gait cycle, side (A) and frontal (B) views. The shorter right step length can be noted by comparing tracings labeled "foot-strike" and "opposite foot-strike." (See Fig. 5.1 for abbreviations.)

5.2A). Pain in the left lower extremity was responsible for an increase in double support and limitation in opposite step length. The greater step length achieved during swing of the painful limb contrasted with the shorter step length achieved during swing phase of the unimpaired limb. Shorter swing phase and earlier application of weight to the sound limb reduced the load on the impaired limb. No new information was added by the frontal view (Fig. 5.2B).

The cadence and walking velocity of this 10-year-old child were comparable to average values for a 7-year-old. Significant asymmetry was evident in duration of single stance. The left lower extremity

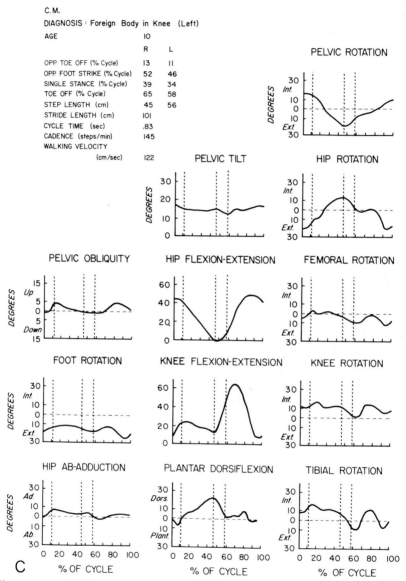

Figure 5.2. (C) Patient C.M. Joint angle curves throughout gait cycle, left lower extremity; frontal, sagittal and transverse planes. No gross abnormalities are noted.

showed single-stance duration of 34% compared with 39% on the right (Fig. 5.2C.). This reduction in single stance was related to the reduction in opposite step length (45 cm right, and 56 cm left) (Fig. 5.2C). The overall gait assessment was that of a mild limp caused by left knee pain. There was insufficient alteration of movement to note movement abnormality in the knee flexion/extension curve (Fig. 5.2C). For this reason another painful anatomical site in the left lower extremity could have produced a similar gait pattern. The patient's complaints of knee pain and swelling were crucial elements in making the diagnosis.

LEGG-CALVÉ-PERTHES DISEASE

M.R., a 6-year-old boy, developed painless limp at age 3½ years. After several months the limp became worse, and he began to complain of right knee pain. Radiographs revealed changes in the femoral head consistent with Legg-Perthes disease, Catterall Grade IV (3). Following hospitalization and traction an arthrogram was performed and containment treatment was started, using a Boston hip orthosis.

Because of the early age of onset of the disease and the beneficial effects of containment (5), the healing process occurred without loss of motion and with relatively normal reconstitution of the femoral head.

The brace was worn for 17 months, and subsequent follow-up examination confirmed a good clinical result. The gait study from which the film tracings and gait data were derived was performed 1½ years after treatment was started. The limp was quite subtle at that time. Nonetheless, the manifestations did not differ significantly from those observed early in the disease process.

A gluteus medius lurch produced by Legg-Calvé-Perthes disease is difficult to identify in the sagittal plane view. In this subject, there was no asymmetry of stepping and no significant change in hip, knee, or ankle posture throughout the gait cycle (Fig. 5.3A). By contrast, the frontal view is highly informative (Fig. 5.3B). The lateral shift of the trunk over the involved hip is apparent (FS to OFS). This shift is a natural protective mechanism brought into play by hip joint pain. The line of application of the floor reaction force is brought closer to the hip joint center, reducing the need for stabilizing action by the hip abductor muscles. This lateral movement of the trunk during single-limb support was first accurately described by Trendelenburg (8) and is frequently called the Trendelenburg gait. When both hips are involved, there is characteristic sway or waddle. This gait abnormality is not specific and may be seen in gluteus medius weakness, hip pain, congenital coxa vara, and congenital dislocation of the hip. A similar trunk sway can also be seen in disorders below the hip joint such as Blount's disease and varus instability of the ankle. In each case, the mechanism is similar, although the cause may be variable. The line of application of the floor reaction force is moved in a more lateral

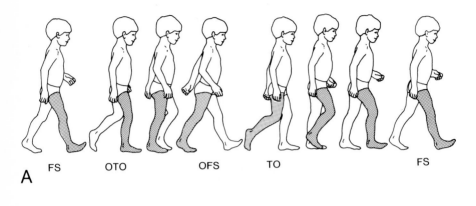

A   FS   OTO   OFS   TO   FS

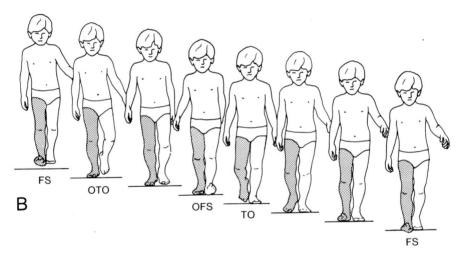

B

FS
OTO
OFS
TO
FS

Figure 5.3. (A and B) Patient M.R.: Legg-Calvé-Perthes disease, right hip. (A) Following period of containment. (B) Frontal plane. Gait cycle begins on the left of the figure. Note the shift of torso and right upper extremity stance phase. (See Fig. 5.1 for abbreviations.)

direction to offer greater stability or relief from pain. It is seen most frequently in hip diseases. A common misconception is that such a movement is pathognomonic of hip disease. Studies in this laboratory have documented occasional cases of "pseudo-Trendelenburg gait."

There was no gross alteration of symmetry in single stance or in step length. Walking velocity and cadence were comparable to the average values for age (Fig. 5.3C). Movement abnormalities were not apparent in the sagittal plane movements of the hip, knee and ankle (Fig. 5.3C). In the transverse plane there was greater than normal external rotation of the hip throughout the cycle.

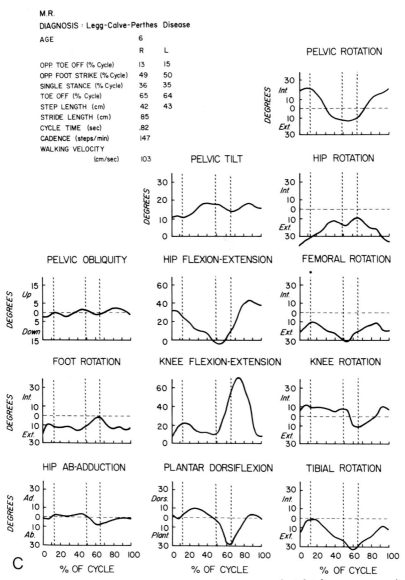

Figure 5.3. (C) Patient M.R. Joint angle curves of right lower extremity, frontal, sagittal and transverse planes.

There were only minor differences in the force curves in the sound left limb and the involved right limb. The principal differences were slight reduction of the second peak (push-off phase) of the vertical force on the right and slight increase of the first peak (loading portion) of the left vertical force curve (Fig. 3D). The combination of vertical

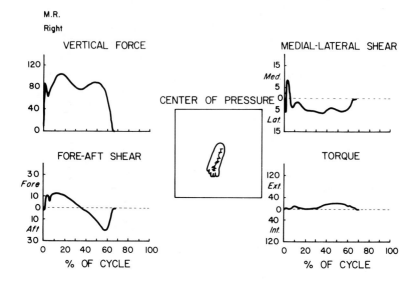

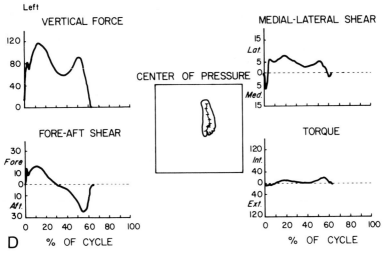

Figure 5.3. (D) Patient M.R. The second peak of the right vertical force is below normal. The first peak of the left vertical force (normal limb) is exaggerated.

force and medial/lateral shear to construct the line of application of the floor reaction force in the frontal plane would have given more information, but this was not done in this instance. Examples of such calculations appear in Chapter 6.

NONSPECIFIC SYNOVITIS OF THE HIP

Patient J.C., a 7-year-old girl, was admitted to Children's Hospital with a 1-week history of right hip pain. Initially, the pain was vague and transitory and there was no obvious limp. Twenty-four hours prior to hospital admission the pain recurred and an antalgic limp was present.

The physical finding on admission was some guarding of movement of the right hip without gross limitation of hip motion. The primary loss of movement was in internal rotation and abduction of the hip. Temperature was normal. WBC 8.7/thousand; differential: neutrophils 59, eosinophils 2, lymphocytes 36, monocytes 3. Sedimentation rate was 18 mm per hour. Radiographs of the hip were entirely normal. On the basis of the clinical findings and history, a diagnosis of nonspecific synovitis of the hip was made and bed rest was ordered (6). The symptoms subsided quickly and the patient was discharged after 2 days of hospitalization. Although a bone scan was not obtained on this patient, one should be ordered because a small number of patients with these symptoms have early Legg-Perthes disease. Limited radio-isotope uptake in the femoral head is the earliest objective marker which can be found in Legg-Perthes disease (2). The radioisotope uptake in the femoral head is usually normal in nonspecific synovitis.

The right hip remained in flexion throughout the gait cycle (Fig. 5.4A). The hip flexion posture was normal at foot-strike, but the usual extension of the hip in stance phase did not follow (OFS) (Fig. 5.4A). The trunk and arms shifted laterally over the painful hip (FS to OFS) (Fig. 5.4B). The lateral movement of the trunk moved the line of application of the floor reaction force closer to the hip joint center, reducing the load on the hip abductor muscles. Through this mechanism the hip joint reaction force was diminished with reduction in hip pain.

There was no difference in duration of single stance, but the step lengths were asymmetrical (Fig. 5.4C). Left step length (contralateral) was 37 cm while the right step length (ipsilateral) was 43 cm. Movements of the involved lower extremity as viewed from the side were abnormal. There was an increased excursion of the pelvic tilt and the hip remained in flexion throughout the gait cycle, with the knee remaining flexed in stance phase and failing to extend in the usual manner (Fig. 5.4C). In addition to these movement abnormalities, hip abduction increased in stance phase.

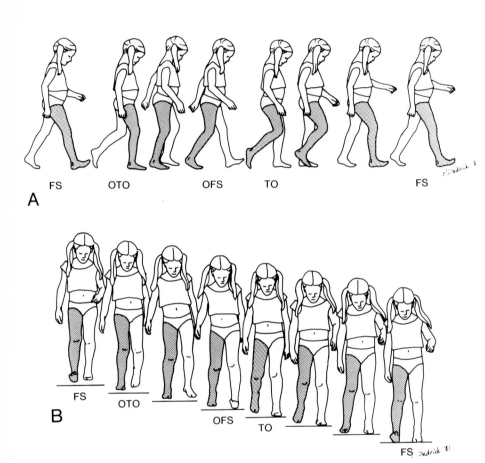

Figure 5.4. (*A* and *B*) Patient J.C.: nonspecific synovitis, right hip. (*A*) Sagittal plane, right gait cycle. Note lack of extension of hip during stance phase. (*B*) Right gait cycle, beginning on the left of the figure. Lateral shift of upper trunk and arm are seen during right stance phase. This abnormal movement is compensatory for hip pain or hip abductor muscle weakness. (See Fig. 5.1 for abbreviations.)

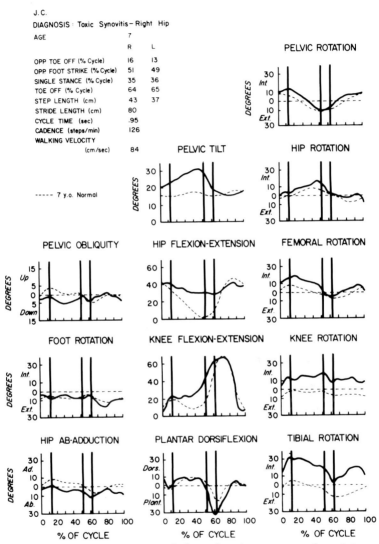

Figure 5.4. (C) Patient J.C. Sagittal, frontal and transverse plane joint angle curves. The *dotted line* represents normal average for age 7. The most obvious movement abnormalities were: exaggerated anterior pelvic tilt, loss of hip extension in stance phase, loss of normal knee extension during single-limb support.

SUMMARY

Limping is defined as relative shortening of single support time due to pain or instability of the weight-bearing limb. It is most clearly recognized as an alteration in the timing of stepping, readily identified in the rapid movement of the opposite swinging limb. Individual case reports of common occult limps have been given. Many common causes of limping have been omitted–for example, the toddler's limp due to unrecognized fracture of the tibia, and the hip limp of an adolescent with slipped capital femoral epiphysis. The differentiation between the limp due to pain and the limp due to muscle paralysis can be made by muscle strength testing, determination of the range of motion, and careful palpation. Formal gait analysis is usually not required to localize the pain site. Inhibition of movement occurs during the walk cycle and helps the observer to pinpoint the problem. Proper identification of limps is a subject of much importance to clinicians.

References

1. Bianco AJ: Juvenile rheumatoid arthritis and ankylosing spondylitis. In Lovell WM, Winter RB: *Pediatric Orthopedics*. Philadelphia, J.B. Lippincott, 1978, Vol I, p 454.
2. Calver R, Venugopal V, Dorgan J, et al: Radionuclide scanning in the early diagnosis of Perthes' disease. *J Bone Joint Surg* 63B:379–382, 1981.
3. Catterall A: The natural history of Perthes disease. *J Bone Joint Surg* 53B:37–53, 1971.
4. Menelaus MB: Discitis. *J Bone Joint Surg* 46B:16–23, 1964.
5. Petrie JG, Bitenc I: The abduction weight-bearing treatment in Legg-Perthes disease. *J Bone Joint Surg* 53B:54–62, 1971.
6. Salter RB: Inflammatory disorders of bones and joints. In *Textbook of Disorders and Injuries of the Musculoskeletal System*. Baltimore, Williams & Wilkins, 1970, pp 186–187.
7. Spiegel PG, Kengla KW, Isaacson AS, et al: Intervertebral disc-space inflammation in children. *J Bone Joint Surg* 54A:284–296, 1972.
8. Trendelenburg F: Über den gang bei angelborener huftselenksluxation. *Dtsch Wochenschr* 2:21–24, 1924.

CHAPTER 6

Congenital Joint Abnormalities

INTRODUCTION

Congenital malformations result from an insult to the embryo in the first trimester of pregnancy and produce errors in formation of the organ or part. An example of this is tibial amelia as noted in Chapter 7. Congenital deformations are related to molding in the last trimester of pregnancy and are thus abnormalities of previously formed parts (4). Dunn (4) described seven postural deformities: facial deformities, plagiocephaly, mandibular asymmetry, sternomastoid torticollis, scoliosis (postural), congenital dislocation of the hip, and talipes. He found statistical correlation in the occurrence of these deformities, emphasizing the need of careful search for the other six when one postural deformity is encountered. Oligohydramnios, first pregnancies, and breech presentation increase chances of congenital birth deformity.

The difference in management of congenital deformations as opposed to congenital malformations is dramatic. With appropriate early treatment, congenital deformations can be brought back to normal alignment and function. In contrast, congenital malformations can never resume normal form or function, because important tissues are missing. Gait abnormalities represented in this chapter are in children with deformations due to congenital dislocation of one or both hips, and congenital clubfoot. If both of these conditions receive early treatment, walking can be normal. Accordingly, cases with delayed or no treatment have been reviewed in order to illustrate typical gait disorders.

CONGENITAL DISLOCATION OF THE HIP

The incidence of hip instability at birth was estimated by Barlow (1) to be 1 in 60. He found that 60% of these infants recover in the first week of life, and 88% in the first 2 months. The remaining infants had true dislocations which persisted unless treated, with an incidence of 1.55/1000.

Von Rosen (21) popularized infant screening for congenital hip dislocation and splinting for all infants with hip instability at birth. According to Von Rosen, late diagnosis and the need for complex orthopaedic surgery were nearly eliminated in Mälmo, Sweden, by early detection and immediate splinting. Further follow-up of the Mälmo experience by Fredensborg (5) supported Von Rosen's conclusion that early detection and treatment lead to normal hip development.

Additional confirmation of the value of careful screening and early treatment was found in a report from Naval Regional Medical Center in San Diego, California (10). Within 72 hours of birth, 15,149 infants were examined over a 4-year period, and the incidence of new hip instability was 0.97%. All of the patients with hip instability were treated from birth and achieved normal hip development. A semirigid abductor brace (Camp brace) was used. No avascular necrosis of the femoral head was observed. Excluding three cases of teratologic dislocations, the surgical rate was 0.01% (two adductor tenotomies).

Other authors have reported less favorable results due to failure of diagnosis or avascular necrosis complicating treatment (7, 22). How can these disparate reports of screening program results be explained? Experiences with a number of screening programs will be required before definitive answers can be given. A review of the literature suggests, however, that primary physicians are the screening physicians in those reports which give the highest failure rate of detection. Diagnostic skill varies from one physician to another, and the most successful screening programs have involved a small number of specially trained individuals to make the diagnosis. With constant practice, their skills have been perfected, and the rate of missed diagnosis is low. This approach is best where a large number of babies are born in one hospital. Implementation of the Mälmo screening model would be difficult in rural settings or communities where there are many small obstetrical units and/or home deliveries. Each community must seek its own solution based upon the local profile of delivering medical services (13).

The relative ease of treating congenital hip dislocation after early detection contrasts sharply with problems in management when diagnosis is delayed. If hip instability is missed at birth, adduction contracture of the hip gradually develops. The Ortolani or Barlow tests which are often positive at birth slowly disappear, due to development of the adduction contracture which prevents reduction. Physical examination reveals shortening, pistoning, and asymmetry of inguinal and buttock folds. There is radiographic evidence of hip dysplasia, subluxation or dislocation.

If the child reaches walking age without treatment, there is a characteristic gait disorder. In a classic paper, Trendelenburg (19) observed that the upper trunk sways toward the side on which the patient puts weight. Movement of the pelvis does not follow trunk motion, but drops to the walking side in distinction from the trunk which moves to the standing side. Trendelenburg correctly deduced that insufficiency of the hip abductor muscles caused the sway. This insufficiency resulted from the change in length and direction of the hip abductor muscles. He recognized that a similar type of gait was found in patients with Duchenne muscular dystrophy. He also described a test to determine the competency of the hip abductors. With the patient standing on the involved leg alone, the opposite buttock should remain level with or above the buttock of the standing leg. Trendelenburg proposed that the measure of success in surgery was related to the function of the abductors as determined by this test. He also concluded that only repositioning of the hip in the acetabulum could ensure successful return of hip abductor muscle function. Trendelenburg's observations are central to current understanding of the subject.

Patient J.S. was the product of a normal pregnancy and was delivered by Cesarean section because of increased fetal size. Her birthweight was 9 pounds, 10 ounces. No abnormalities were noted at birth, and she began to walk at 10½ months. Her growth and development seemed normal, but at 5 years of age, she was referred to an orthopaedic surgeon because of left intoeing. The orthopaedist observed signs of right hip abnormality and ordered x-rays which revealed right congenital hip dislocation (Fig. 6.1, A and B).

On examination, short-leg gait with mild right gluteus medius limp was noted. Galeazzi's sign was positive on the right, but Ortolani's sign was negative. Ranges of motion in the hips were:

	Right	Left
Flexion	140	140
Extension	0	0
Internal rotation	65	55
External rotation	50	40
Abduction	40	60
Adduction	30	30

There was no pistoning of the hip. According to the family, the patient had been a toe-walker from the first year, as well as an in-toer on the left side.

The advanced dysplasia of the acetabulum required extensive realignment to restore joint stability. The neck shaft angle of the femur was 130° and the anteversion was 32° (Fig. 6.1C). The surgical plan for the femur was to shorten without significant change in the femoral geometry. Open reduction of the right hip, capsulorrhaphy, Salter osteotomy (15), femoral shortening, adductor release, and iliopsoas recession were performed under a single anesthetic as one-stage reconstruction (12) (Fig. 6.1D).

In a preoperative gait study, tracings of film from the right side camera suggested shortening of the right lower extremity (Fig. 6.1G). Tracings of the front camera film showed marked drop of the contralateral iliac crest at the beginning of single-limb support (opposite toe-

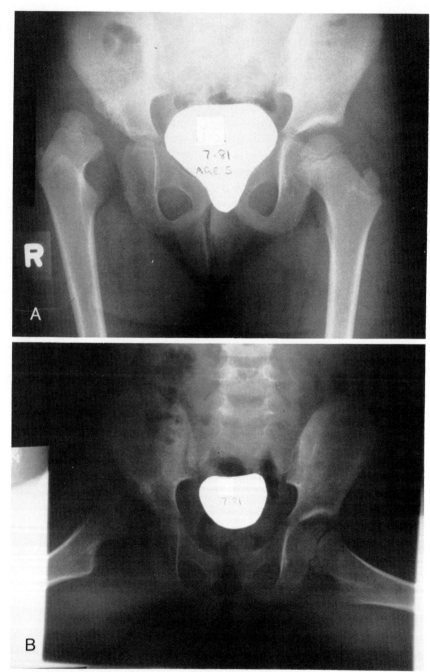

Figure 6.1. (*A* and *B*) Patient J.S.: Congenital abnormality. (*A*) Untreated right congenital hip subluxation with false acetabulum. (*B*) Frog view of hips.

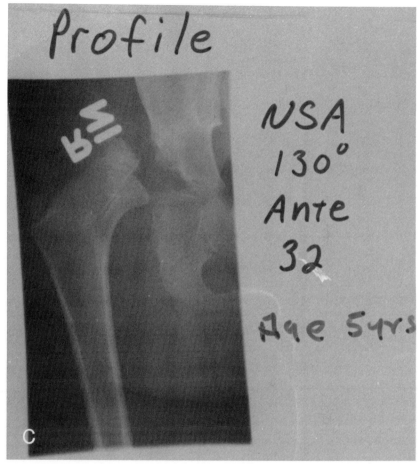

Figure 6.1. (C) Patient J.S. Profile view of right hip taken during fluoroscopic study for anteversion and neck shaft angle. Anteversion measured 32° and neck shaft angle, 130°.

off). Shift of the shoulder over the right hip was apparent in comparing opposite toe-off and toe-off (Fig. 6.1*I*). These are the components of a gluteus medius lurch. Ordinarily the arm is held in abduction during single-limb stance, but in this case, the child held both hands in front of her. Postoperative tracings of film from the right side camera show increased step length and normal reciprocal arm and leg movements (Fig. 6.1*H*).

Tracings of film from the front camera taken postoperatively demonstrated reduction in the gluteus medius lurch and correction of the marked drop of the left iliac crest during right single-limb support (Fig. 6.1*J*). Walking velocity and reduction of cadence were improved in

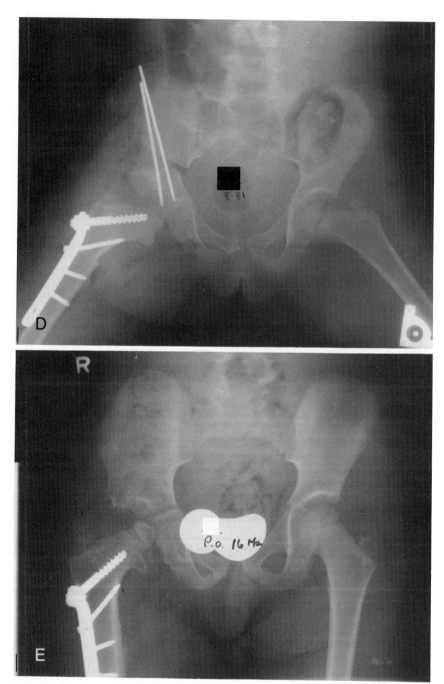

Figure 6.1.   (*D* and *E*) Patient J.S. after one-stage reconstruction of the hip (*D*) and 16 months postoperatively (*E*).

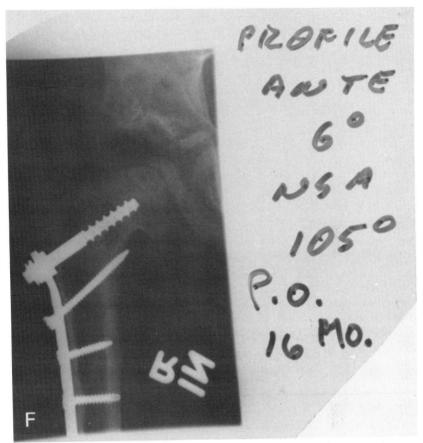

Figure 6.1. (F) Patient J.S. Profile view taken during fluoroscopic study to determine postoperative anteversion and neck shaft angle.

the postoperative study. Stride length increased from 73 cm before surgery to 90 cm afterward (Fig. 6.1K).

Movement abnormalities of the right lower extremity in the preoperative study included increased internal rotation of the pelvis, increased external rotation of the femur, and exaggerated external rotation of the hip (Fig. 6.1K). Changes following surgery included increases in internal rotation of the pelvis and external rotation of the hip joint.

Although the overall effect upon gait was beneficial and joint stability was evident (Fig. 6.1E), the postoperative gait study and assessment of femoral anteversion and neck shaft angle indicated unsatisfactory femoral alignment (anteversion, 6°, and neck shaft angle, 105°) (Fig. 6.1F).

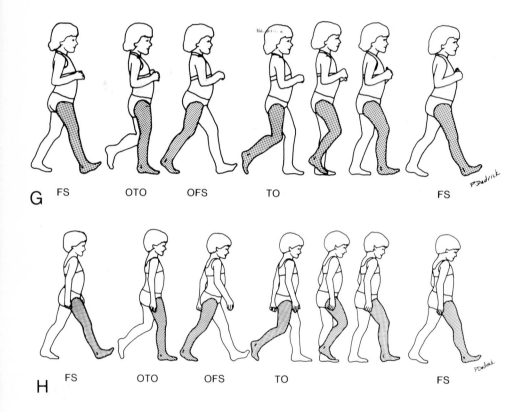

Figure 6.1. (G and H) Patient J.S. Tracings of right camera film, preoperative (G) and postoperative (H). (FS = foot-strike, OTO = opposite toe-off, OFS = opposite foot-strike, and TO = toe-off.)

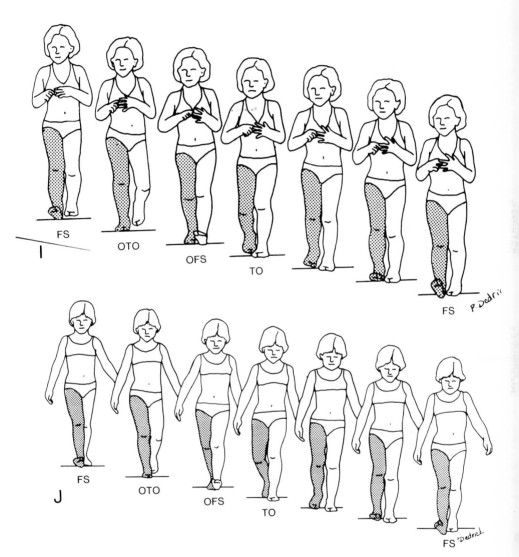

Figure 6.1. (*I* and *J*) Patient J.S. Tracings of front camera film, preoperative (*I*) and postoperative (*J*).

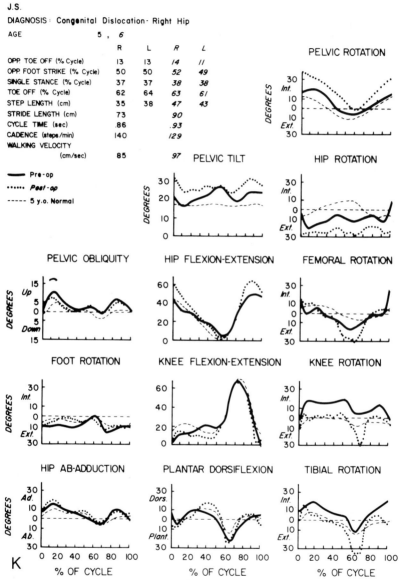

Figure 6.1. (K) Patient J.S. Preoperative and postoperative linear measurements and joint angle rotations, right lower extremity. Joint angle rotations are compared with values for 5-year-old normal subjects.

This patient now has a transverse plane movement abnormality which is due to coxa vara alignment of the hip and absence of normal anteversion. The Salter procedure diminished internal rotation of the hip, adding to the effect of excessive femoral derotation osteotomy. Options are to await further bony remodeling of the hip with probable improvement of the neck shaft angle, or realign the femur to approximately 20° of anteversion and 120° of neck shaft angle. This alignment would correct the present transverse plane motion abnormality. The neck shaft angle frequently increases spontaneously when overcorrection is carried out. However, it is unlikely that any improvement in rotation of the femur will take place without surgery. The child is asymptomatic at this time, and the parents are considering the recommendation for additional surgery to restore optimal alignment.

Patient M.C., a 7-year-old child, was referred by a chiropractor for treatment of bilateral hip dislocations. According to the mother, the dislocations were detected at 3 years of age. The parents sought advice from many doctors, but no treatment plan was begun. Over the 2 years preceding examination, chiropractic manipulations were done with no noticeable change.

Examination revealed a 7-year-old child who walked with the classic lordotic waddling gait of bilateral hip dislocations. The trunk sway was both lateral and posterior, and the thighs were markedly shortened. Hip ranges of motion were:

	Right	Left
Flexion	90	90
Extension	0	0
Abduction	45	45
Internal rotation	45	45
External rotation	90	90

There was bilateral pistoning of the hips, but a negative Ortolani test. X-rays showed bilateral high gluteal dislocations (Fig. 6.2A).

The risks are great with bilateral congenital hip dislocation surgery undertaken at this age. Age 5 or 6 is considered the upper limit for these procedures. When both hips are involved above this age limit, significant residual stiffness in one hip may develop, causing asymmetrical gait and premature onset of pain.

The treatment carried out for this child is controversial because of her age at the time of surgery. One-stage open reduction, capsulorrhaphy, double innominate osteotomy, femoral shortening, adductor release, and iliopsoas recession were performed on the right, and 6 months later on the left (12, 18) (Fig. 6.2, B and C). The patient has regained good motion and stability on the right and is recovering motion on the left, but insufficient time has elapsed to allow proper evaluation.

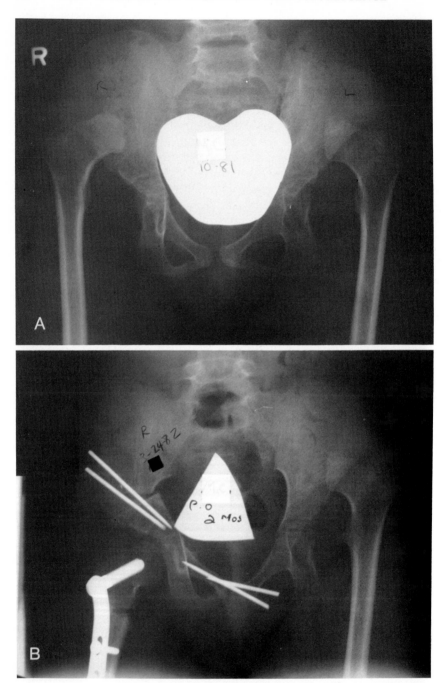

Figure 6.2. (*A* and *B*) Patient M.C.: congenital abnormality. (*A*) Bilateral congenital dislocation of the hip, age 7 years. (*B*) At 2 months following one-stage reconstruction of the hip.

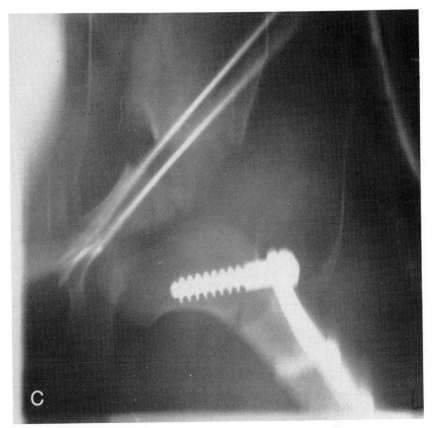

Figure 6.2. (C) Patient M.C. immediately following one-stage reconstruction of left hip.

In a preoperative gait study, tracings of film from the side camera revealed lordotic posture and posterior alignment of the arms in stance phase (Fig. 6.2D). The upper thigh segments were shortened, producing disproportion between the upper and lower segments of the lower extremities, secondary to the hip dislocations. Preoperative tracings from the front camera film showed bilateral gluteus medius lurch (Fig. 6.2E).

Linear measurements were: cadence, 145 steps per minute; walking velocity, 100 cm per second. Joint angle measurements were compared with adult normals (Fig. 6.2F). Abnormalities included excessive anterior pelvic tilt, excessive hip flexion, loss of knee flexion wave in stance phase, absent pelvic rotation, and increased external rotation of the foot. Force measurements of the right lower extremity showed diminished second peak vertical force, and diminished forward and aft shear (Fig. 6.2G). The left lower extremity force measurements showed impaired loading, delayed aft shear and absent torque.

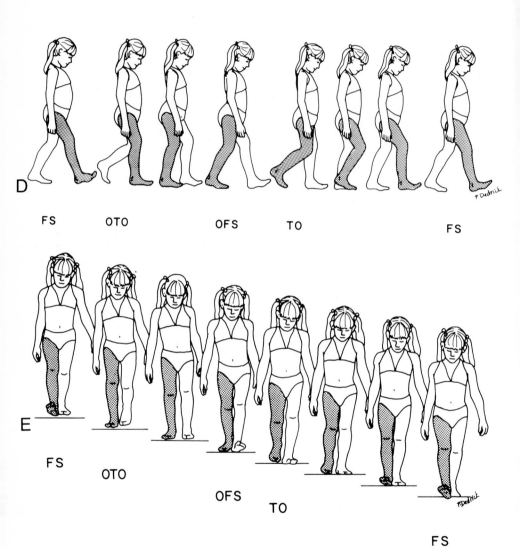

Figure 6.2.   (*D* and *E*) Patient M.C. Preoperative film tracings from right side (*D*) and front (*E*) camera. (See Fig. 6.1 for abbreviations.)

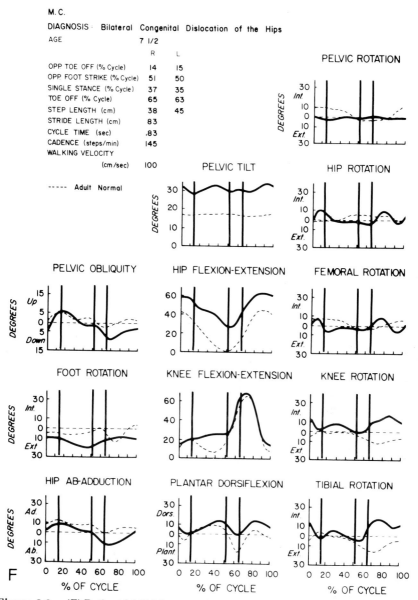

Figure 6.2. (F) Patient M.C. Linear measurements and joint angle rotations— preoperative. The joint angle rotations are compared with adult normal.

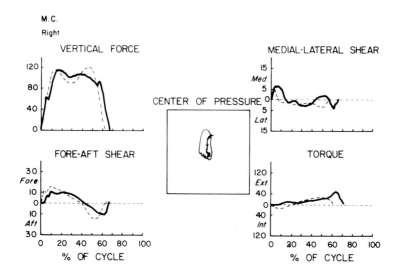

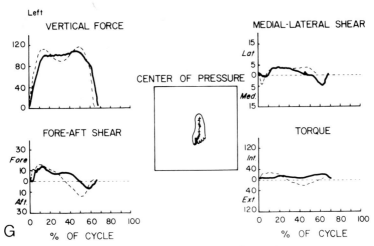

Figure 6.2.   (G) Patient M.C. Preoperative force plate measurements.

CONGENITAL CLUBFOOT

Congenital idiopathic clubfoot is defined as a congenital birth defect characterized by equinus contracture at the ankle, inversion of the hind foot, and supination and inversion of the forefoot. It is not to be confused with similar deformities with known etiology—for example, paralytic clubfoot in myelomeningocele. The incidence of this defect in the general population is approximately 1 in 1000 live births (17). The sex ratio is 2.17 to 1, male to female. The chances that a second child in the family will have the deformity are increased more than 20 times (1 in 35) (23). McKusick (11) states that, although genetic factors are clearly important, simple inheritance has not been established.

Antonio Scarpa (14) in 1818 described the primary problem in clubfoot as that of deformity of the talus. This emphasis was gradually forgotten, and anomalous tendon insertions and abnormal muscle pulls were described as causative factors in production of the clubfoot (17). Irani and Sherman (6) dissected 11 extremities in stillbirths or neonatal deaths and studied 14 completely normal controls, reporting no primary abnormalities in vessels, nerves, muscles or tendon insertions in the clubfoot. Settle (16) came to the same conclusion in a similar study which also included histological study of the spinal cord. The extreme conservative treatment with no surgery from former years (8, 9) has now been replaced by recommended early operation for all infants or children not responding to stretching and casting. The posteromedial release developed by Turco (20), or some modification of this (3), can be used from infancy to approximately 4 years of age to effect correction. Early complete surgical correction reduces the chance of recurrence and the need for multiple operations.

Patient R.V. was born with a left congenital clubfoot. Casting of the foot was done from 1 to 3 months of age in Mexico, but the foot deformity persisted. The patient began to walk at 15 months and subsequently appeared to do well in spite of a limp and obvious deformity of the foot. He was first seen at 4 years of age in the Orthopedic Clinic at San Diego Children's Hospital.

Abnormal musculoskeletal findings were limited to the left lower extremity. A marked talipes equinovarus deformity could not be brought into corrected position. Iowa frame x-ray views revealed parallelism of the talus and calcaneus on anteroposterior and lateral views with a Beatson index of 25° (Fig. 6.3, A and B). This low index indicated severe clubfoot. Gait study was performed when the patient was 4 years old. Film tracings from the side camera showed inverted foot and ankle equinus (Fig. 6.3E). Film tracings from the front camera showed an inverted foot with fixed varus (Fig. 6.3F). The foot contacted the floor on the extreme lateral edge and dorsum of the foot.

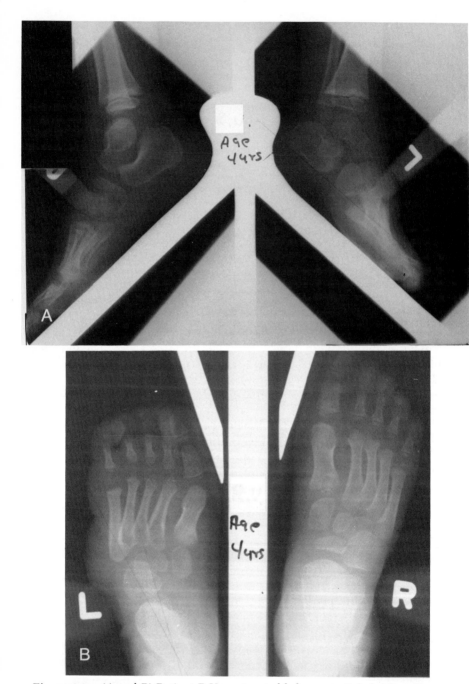

Figure 6.3. (*A* and *B*) Patient R.V.: untreated left congenital clubfoot. Preoperative lateral (*A*) and AP (*B*) views of both feet in Iowa frame.

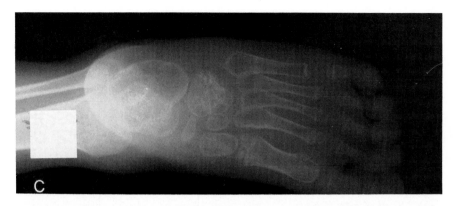

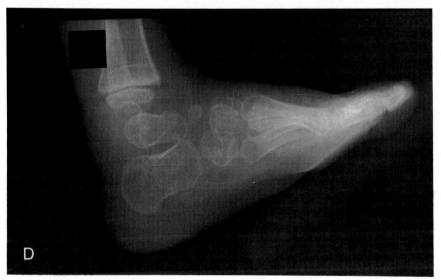

Figure 6.3. (*C* and *D*) Patient R.V. X-rays 11 months postoperatively, AP (*C*) and lateral (*D*) views.

Walking velocity was 52 cm, cadence, 111, and stride length, 56, compared with the normal of 87 cm, 154 and 67, respectively. Single stance was restricted on the left (29%) (Fig. 6.3*G*).

The joint angle rotations of the left lower extremity were compared with the 3-year-old normal values (Fig. 6.3*G*). Ankle plantar flexion-dorsiflexion could not be measured because of the extreme deformity. Exaggerated external rotation was noted in both pelvic and femoral rotation. In spite of this, the foot was internally rotated 30° throughout the cycle.

Force plate measurements revealed impaired loading on the right and diminished aft shear (Fig. 6.3*H*). The center of pressure progression was relatively normal. Force plate measurements for the left lower

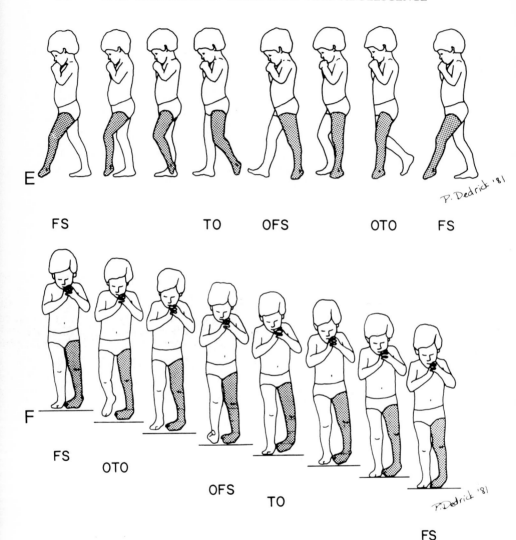

Figure 6.3.   (*E* and *F*) Patient R.V. Preoperative film tracings from left side (*E*) and front (*F*) camera. (See Fig. 6.1 for abbreviations.)

extremity demonstrated impaired loading, diminished forward shear and total concentration of pressure in the mid-lateral portion of the foot.

Electromyograms obtained with surface electrodes of the left peroneals, tibialis anterior and gastrocnemius soleus did not reveal significant alteration in muscle phasic activity by comparison with values for normal 4-year-olds. The swing phase activity in the normal gastrocnemius soleus was present in only 7 of 37 normal subjects (Fig. 6.3*I*).

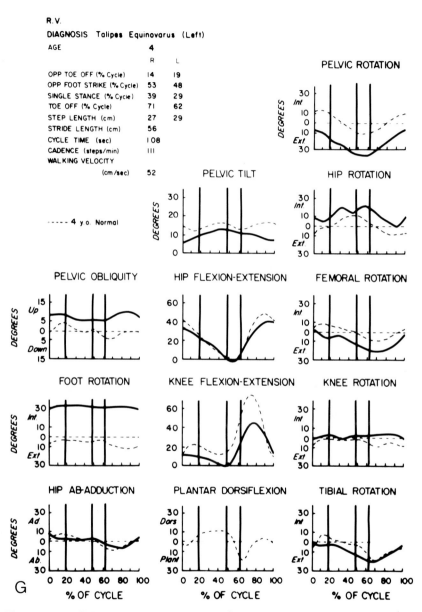

Figure 6.3. (G) Patient R.V. Preoperative linear measurements and joint angle rotations, left lower extremity. Joint angle rotations are compared with values for 4-year-old normal subjects.

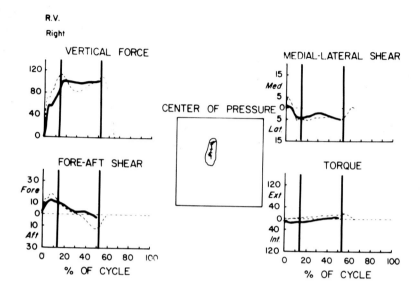

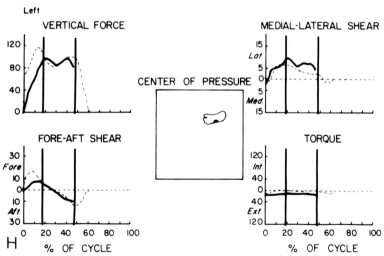

Figure 6.3.   (*H*) Patient R.V. Preoperative force plate measurements compared with normal 4-year-old subjects. Force recording is incomplete because the opposite foot contacted the same force plate.

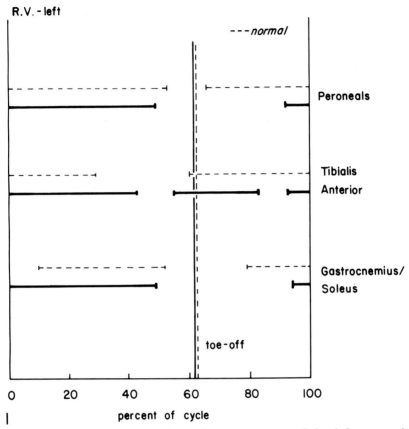

Figure 6.3. (*I*) Patient R.V. Phase electromyograms of the left peroneals, tibialis anterior and gastrocnemius soleus with 4-year-old normal subject for comparison. The normal subjects had inconstant swing phase activity in the gastrocnemius soleus.

Summary of the gait analysis indicated a primary movement abnormality (constant internal rotation, equinus, and supination of the left foot, with concentration of weight bearing on the dorsal and lateral edge of the foot throughout stance phase). Compensation was good, as expected with a single-level defect and intact control system. A limp was present, manifested by diminished single stance. External rotation of the pelvis and femur partially compensated for the severe internal rotation of the foot. Because of difficulties in obtaining appropriate shoes, the presence of a limp, cosmetic factors, and anticipated future problems related to altered weight bearing, surgery was performed to realign the foot.

The surgery included posteromedial release and cuboid decancellation. Good correction was achieved and 11 months later, the child could walk and run without a limp. The foot was plantigrade. The heel was in neutral alignment, and the ankle could be brought into 10° of dorsiflexion (Fig. 6.3, C and D). This was considered an excellent surgical result in view of the child's age at the time of surgery.

References

1. Barlow TG: Early diagnosis and treatment of congenital dislocation of the hip. *J Bone Joint Surg* 44B:292–301, 1962.
2. Beatson TR, Pearson JR: A method of assessing correction in clubfoot. *J Bone Joint Surg* 48B:40–50, 1966.
3. Carroll NS, McMurtry R, Leete SF: The pathoanatomy of congenital clubfoot. *Orthop. Clin. North Am* 9:225–232, 1978.
4. Dunn PM: Congenital postural deformities. *Br Med Bull* 32:71–76, 1976.
5. Fredensborg N: The results of early treatment of typical congenital dislocation of the hip in Mälmo. *J Bone Joint Surg* 58B:272–278, 1976.
6. Irani RN, Sherman MS: The pathologic anatomy of clubfoot. *J Bone Joint Surg* 45A:45–52, 1963.
7. Jones D: An assessment of the value of examination of the hip in the newborn. *J Bone Joint Surg* 59B:318–322, 1977.
8. Kite JH: *The Clubfoot.* New York, Grune & Stratton, 1964.
9. Kite JH: Nonoperative treatment of congenital clubfoot. *Clin Orthop* 84:29–38, 1972.
10. McKinnon B, Bosse MJ, Browning WH: Congenital hip dysplasia; the subluxable variety. *J Pediatr Orthop* 2:214, 1982.
11. McKusick VA: *Mendelian Inheritance in Man*, ed 5. Baltimore, Johns Hopkins University Press, 1978, p 72.
12. Mubarak SJ, Rowe F, Sutherland DH, et al: One-stage procedure for the correction of untreated congenital dislocation of the hip in the older child (abstract submitted to Pediatric Orthopedic Society, November 1981) (in press).
13. Paterson D: The early diagnosis and screening of congenital dislocation of the hip. In Tachdjian MO: *Congenital Dislocation of the Hip.* New York, Churchill Livingstone, 1982, Ch 5, pp 145–157.
14. Scarpa A: A memoir in the congenital clubfeet of children and mode of correcting that deformity. Translated from the Italian by J. H. Wishart. Edinburgh, A. Constable and Company, 1918.
15. Salter RB: Innominate osteotomy in the treatment of congenital dislocation and subluxation of the hip. *J Bone Joint Surg* 43B:518–539, 1961.
16. Settle GW: The anatomy of congenital talipes equinovarus: sixteen dissected specimens. *J Bone Joint Surg* 45A:1341–1354, 1963.
17. Stewart SF: Clubfoot—its incidence and treatment. *J Bone Joint Surg* 33A:477–589, 1951.
18. Sutherland DH, Greenfield R: Double innominate osteotomy. *J Bone Joint Surg* 59A:1082–1091, 1977.
19. Trendelenburg F: Concerning gait in congenital dislocation of the hip. *Dtsch Med Wochenschr* 21:22–24, 1895.
20. Turco V: Surgical correction of the resistant clubfoot. *J Bone Joint Surg* 53A:477–497, 1971.
21. Von Rosen S: Diagnosis and treatment of congenital dislocation of the hip joint in the newborn. *J Bone Joint Surg* 44B:284–291, 1962.
22. Williamson J: Difficulties of early diagnosis and treatment of congenital dislocation of the hip in Northern Ireland. *J Bone Joint Surg* 54B:13–17, 1972.
23. Wynne-Davis R: Family studies and the cause of congenital clubfoot. *J Bone Joint Surg* 46B:445–451, 1964.

CHAPTER 7

Lower Limb Deficiencies

INTRODUCTION

Deficiencies in the lower limb may be primary embryopathic defects or secondary amputations necessitated by a trauma, sepsis, or malignant tumor. Amputation is also performed sometimes for the limb-deficient child to eliminate a poorly functioning segment or to accommodate a good prosthetic fitting.

Classification of congenital limb deficiencies differentiates between transverse and longitudinal defects and further subdivides into terminal and intercalary defects (6). (The latter term refers to a deficiency in the middle with normal development above and below.) The terms *amelia* (absence of the limb), *hemimelia* (absence of forearm and hand or leg and foot), and *acheiria or apodia* (absence of hand or foot), *adactylia* (absence of all five digits and their metacarpals or metatarsals), and *aphalangia* (absence of one or more phalanges from all five digits) further complete the classification.

A number of features distinguish the child with congenital amputation from the adult with acquired amputation (1, 8, 9). The child has no memory of a complete body image and thus experiences no grief reaction. Treatment planning must include growth assessment, and prostheses must be constructed frequently to accommodate growth. The energy level of a healthy child is apparently inexhaustible, and the ability to adapt to any prosthetic device borders on the phenomenal.

The child who requires secondary amputation seldom experiences persistent phantom limb sensation which disturbs many adult amputees. Until now, the advantages noted have all been for the child, but one problem remains unique to the child amputee. Below-knee amputations commonly result in terminal overgrowth (1, 8, 9). This produces a bone spike on the distal tibia which can erode the skin. This pencil-shaped growth does not come from an adjacent open epiphysis, but from an appositional bone growth (9). Below-knee amputation should be avoided whenever possible, because of the high incidence of terminal overgrowth. The site of the ankle joint is preferable, since the presence of articular cartilage in an end-bearing stump eliminates this complication. For this reason, the Syme amputation is selected, rather than below-knee amputation, if the choice exists (4). Other reasons for choosing the more distal site include the

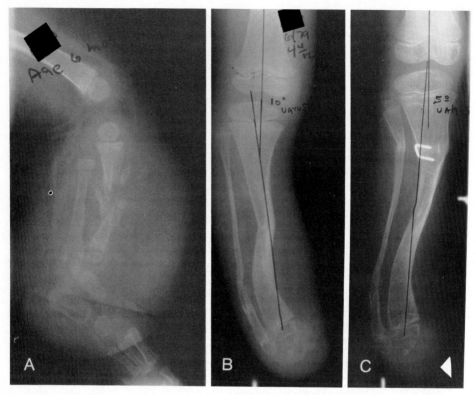

Figure 7.1. (A–C) Patient C.P.: congenital pseudarthrosis of tibia and fibula, and large lipoma, seen at 6 months (A). At 4 years and 4 months (B), healed pseudarthrosis of tibia following Syme amputation. Femoral-tibial angle—10° of varus. (C) Following proximal tibial osteotomy, 5° valgus femoral-tibial angle.

advantages of retaining a longer lever-arm, better end-bearing, and more suitable prosthesis.

Some of the clinical factors which determine how well any amputee walks are: limb length, muscle power, type of end-bearing (bone versus articular cartilage), condition of stump skin, socket fit, prosthetic alignment, prosthetic design, and the training and experience of the prosthetic user.

Three clinical studies will follow this introductory review.

SYME AMPUTATION

Patient C.P. was born with severe pseudarthrosis of the tibia. In addition to a large bone-deficient area in the tibia, the entire calf and ankle were enlarged by a huge lipoma (Fig. 7.1A). Two unsuccessful attempts were made to secure union by excising the fibrous tissue and bone grafting. Staged resection of the lipomatous mass was performed, after multiple biopsies to rule out malignancy. When union was not obtained, Syme amputation was carried out. Following this, a pylon temporary prosthesis allowed immediate ambulation. The elements of the permanent prosthesis were patellar-bearing total contact socket, plastic shank, and SACH foot (solid ankle cushion heel foot) (5, 10).

A gait study was done at 4 years and 10 months of age, because the child had developed varus thrust in the knee and was having difficulty with the suspension system of the prosthesis. (The prosthesis fell off in the middle of play.) X-rays of the tibia showed varus alignment (Fig. 7.1B). After gait analysis, proximal tibial osteotomy restored appropriate tibial alignment, eliminating lateral thrust of the knee during single-limb support, and prosthetic suspension became secure. The tibia healed in good alignment (Fig. 7.1C). A second gait study done 9 months postoperatively was the basis for assessment of changes resulting from surgery. Preoperative film tracings from the side camera

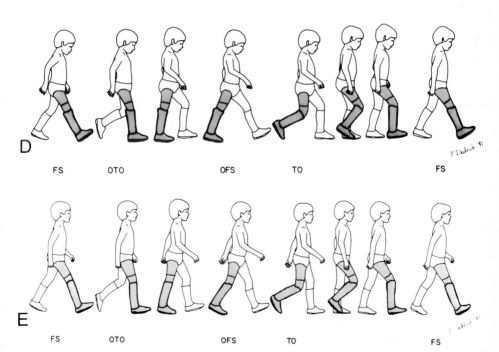

Figure 7.1. (D and E) Patient C.P. Film tracings from right side camera, preoperative (D) and postoperative (E). (FS = foot-strike, OTO = opposite toe-off, OFS = opposite foot-strike, and TO = toe-off.)

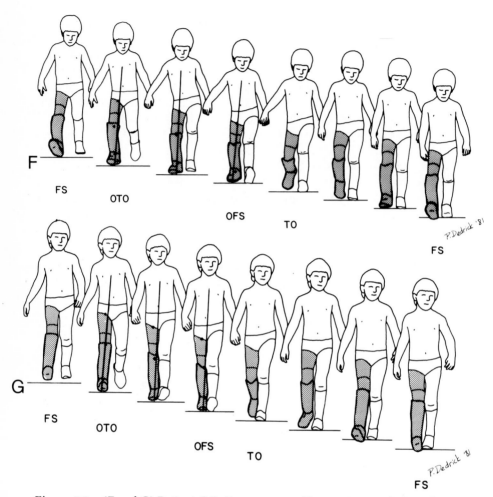

Figure 7.1. (*F* and *G*) Patient C.P. Front camera film tracings with force line superimposed during single-limb support, preoperative (*F*) and postoperative (*G*).

showed quite normal gait with the exception of excessive contralateral knee flexion at toe-off (Fig. 7.1*D*). Preoperative film tracings from the front camera are shown with the force line superimposed during single-limb support (Fig. 7.1*F*). Figure 7.1*E* demonstrates improvement in posture throughout the cycle in side film tracings, and Figure 7.1*G* shows reduction in trunk sway and movement of the force line closer to the knee center during single-limb support. Overall improvement in dynamic posture can be appreciated by comparing film tracings of opposite foot-strike before and after surgery (Fig. 7.1, *F* and *G*). The

C.P. — RIGHT-FRONT TORQUE
MID-STANCE

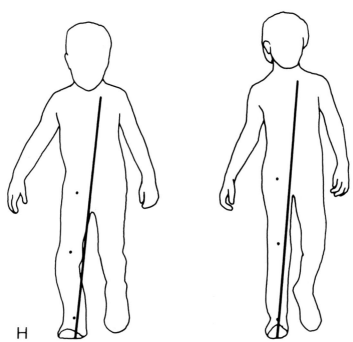

H

Figure 7.1. (*H*) Patient C.P. Comparative film tracings from front camera taken at mid-stance with force line superimposed before and after osteotomy of the proximal right tibia.

contrast is even more dramatic in the comparison at mid-stance (Fig. 7.1*H*). Increased medial deviation of the force line from the knee joint center with excessive compression of the medial growth plate was the probable cause of the progressive varus growth through Heuter-Volkmann's law (7). Reduction of excessive medial compression of the medial growth plate restored more normal tibial growth, and good tibial alignment has remained.

The linear measurements changed only slightly following surgery (Fig. 7.1*I*). Cadence, walking, and velocity were appropriate for age both before and after surgery. The differences in joint angle rotation before and after were most striking in hip, femoral, and knee rotations. During single-limb support, severe external rotation of the femur, external rotation of the hip, and internal rotation of the knee were noted. These changes were also present in patients with Blount's disease and severe physiologic genu varum (see Chapter 4). Following restoration of tibial alignment, more normal hip, femoral, and knee rotations were present.

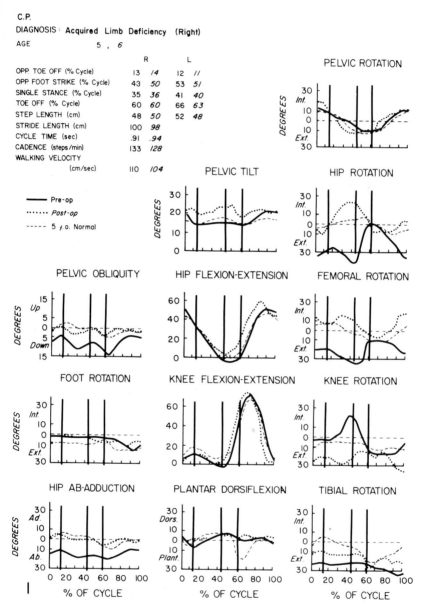

Figure 7.1. (*I*) Patient C.P. Linear measurements and joint angle rotations of right lower extremity before and 9 months after osteotomies of proximal tibia and fibula.

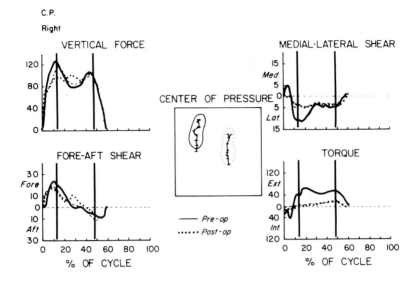

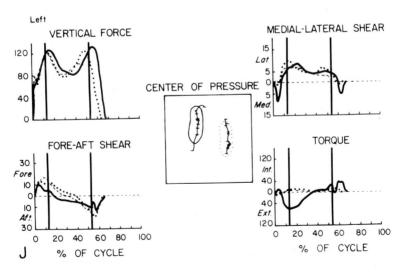

Figure 7.1. (J) Patient C.P. Preoperative and postoperative floor reaction forces of right lower extremity with values for normal 5-year-old subjects for comparison. The *dotted lines* represent the normal values.

The force curves differed only minimally after surgery (Fig. 7.1J). The lateral shear which was excessive at the beginning of single-limb support preoperatively followed a normal pattern postoperatively. The

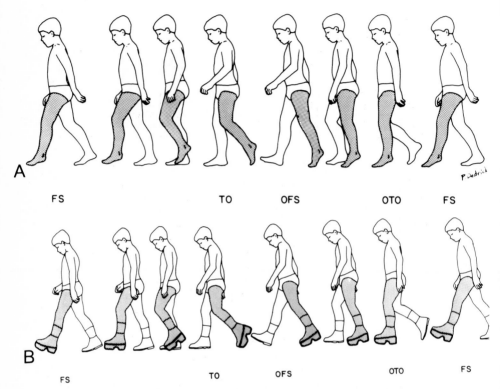

Figure 7.2. (*A* and *B*) Patient S.P.: left lower extremity limb deficiency. Film tracings from side camera (*A*) and with subject wearing shoe buildup (*B*). (See Fig. 7.1 for abbreviations.)

excessive external torque in single-limb support also became normal postoperatively.

The tibia vara deformity has not recurred, and prosthetic alignment and suspension are no longer problematic.

This case illustrates the usefulness of gait analysis in establishing the gait deviations of an amputee with a gait problem and documenting the outcome of treatment.

FEMORAL FOCAL DEFICIENCY

Patient S.P. was born with mild shortening of the left lower extremity. The difference in limb length in infancy was 1.5 cm. The discrepancy increased, requiring shoe lifts of increasing size. At 12½ years of age, the inequality measured 6.4 cm by scanogram, and a large shoe elevation was used. The hip joint was stable, and there was no coxa vara. Hip abduction strength was normal, and no muscle contractures were present. The absence of clinical findings, except the substantial

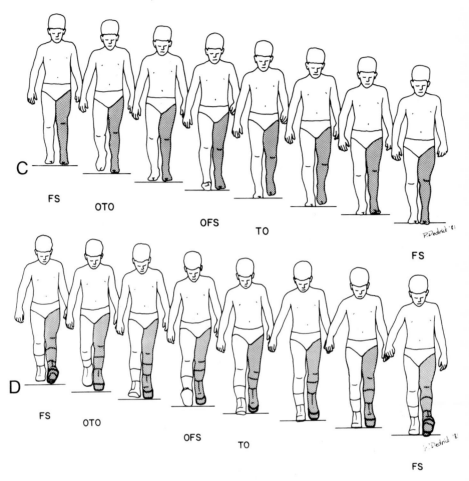

Figure 7.2. (*C* and *D*) Patient S.P. Film tracings from front camera (*C*) and with subject wearing shoe buildup (*D*).

leg length inequality, could indicate an alternate diagnosis of congenital hypoplasia of the lower extremity. The distribution of the leg length inequality (4-cm shortening of the femur, and 2.4 cm in the tibia) supported this diagnosis.

Gait analysis was performed with and without the shoe elevation. Film tracings from the left side camera (Fig. 7.2*A*) showed equinus posture of the left ankle in stance and swing phase. This equinus posture compensated for the short limb during stance phase. The reason for equinus in swing phase is less certain. A plausible explanation is that severe discrepancy eliminated the need for dorsiflexion for foot clearance in swing phase, and the control mechanisms which

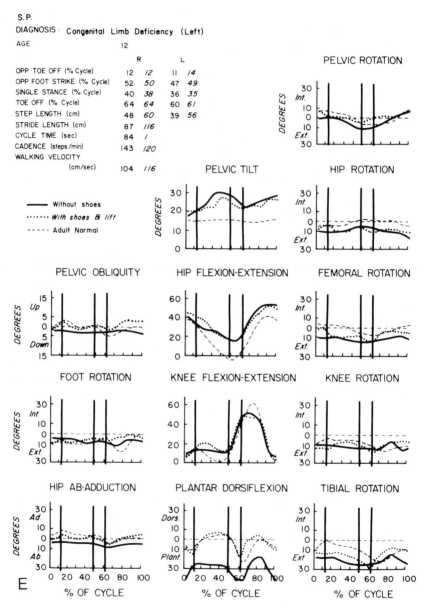

Figure 7.2. (E) Patient S.P. Linear measurements and joint angle rotations with and without use of shoe elevation. Comparison is made with adult normal joint angles.

effect economy of energy expenditure in walking excluded unnecessary muscle action. Tracings of the front film (Fig. 7.2C) show compensation for limb length shortening by equinus posture of the left ankle.

Film tracings from the side camera with the subject wearing shoe elevation show increased left step length, return of heel-strike, and normal ankle dorsiflexion during swing phase (Fig. 7.2B). Presumably, restoration of full limb length by shoe elevation reproduced the necessity for dorsiflexion of the ankle to clear the foot in swing phase.

Restoration of heel-strike is clearly demonstrated in film tracings from the front camera (Fig. 7.2D). The changes in step length and walking velocity were surprising (Fig. 7.2E). Walking velocity with the shoe elevation increased 12% (from 104 to 116 cm per second). Cadence dropped from 143 to 120 steps per minute. The right step length increased 25% from 48 to 60 cm. Left step length increased 44% from 39 to 56 cm.

The changes in joint angle were most evident in ankle plantar flexion/dorsiflexion (Fig. 7.2E). Addition of the shoe lift restored normal ankle motion. The work output fell from 0.672 kcal/kg/km to 0.40 kcal/kg/km with wearing the shoe elevation.

Conclusions drawn from this study were that the lift restored symmetry to walking, increased step length and walking velocity, and improved walking efficiency as measured by work output.

Limb lengthening is reserved for patients with 5 cm or more of shortening, because patients with lesser discrepancies can be treated more safely by retarding growth of the sound limb or by surgical shortening. Two-stage limb lengthening is planned for this patient— the femur first and then the tibia. Problems are anticipated, as limb lengthening is most difficult in patients with congenital shortening.

CONGENITAL RIGHT TERMINAL TIBIAL HEMIMELIA

Patient R.O. was born to a para I, gravida I mother 2½ weeks prematurely. Deformities present at birth included total absence of the right tibia, deformity and medial deficiency of the right foot, and an accessory toe on the medial dorsal aspect of the left foot. The father's cousin was born with bilateral absence of the tibia and the child's father was born with ectrodactyly of the hand and a congenital malformation of the foot.

Both parents were able to freely discuss treatment options from the day following the child's birth. Knee joint disarticulation was recommended because of severe leg length inequality, knee instability, and congenital abnormality of the foot. Other treatment choices were discussed (2), but the family elected to proceed with amputation at the time when walking was attempted.

Standing and attempted cruising began at 9 months and knee joint disarticulation and removal of the left accessory toe were carried out soon thereafter. Figure 7.3A shows an x-ray of the lower extremities before elective knee joint disarticulation. A rigid surgical dressing was applied in the operating room immediately after the amputation, and a temporary pylon was attached during the hospital stay, so that the infant could begin standing. By 12 months of age, the child was wearing a prosthesis without a knee joint, replacing the plaster socket and pylon, and physical therapy gait training began. By 18 months of age, the child was entirely independent in walking, playful, and unconcerned about the prosthesis.

The advantages of early amputation when it appears inevitable are obvious. The deficient limb is removed before the child's body image is fully formed, and there is no grief reaction. If the prosthesis can be applied at a time when walking is developing, the child learns to walk with the friendly prosthesis. The child in this case is happy, well-adjusted, and secure in a loving home, and he will grow up without memories of frequent hospitalizations, multiple surgical procedures, and probable amputation at a more vulnerable age.

A gait study was performed at 2 years of age. Film tracings from the right side camera showed stiff knee gait and vigorous arm swing (Fig. 7.3B). Film tracings from the front camera demonstrated marked circumduction of the leg during swing phase (Fig. 7.3C).

Cadence was 120 steps per minute; walking velocity, 55 cm per second; and stride length, 55, in comparison with the normal for age of 161, 76 cm, and 61 respectively (Fig. 7.3D). Single stance duration on the right was 30 and on the left, 39. These measurements indicated low cadence, normal stride length, and short single stance. Movement measurements showed exaggerated hip flexion in swing phase with marked hip abduction. These movement measurements confirmed the visual appearance of circumduction. The absence of knee motion because of the nonarticulated prosthesis required excessive hip flexion and abduction in swing phase to clear the foot.

Surface electromyograms of the gluteus maximus and gluteus medius revealed stance phase prolongation of the maximus and premature onset of phasic activity in the gluteus medius (Fig. 7.3E). The gluteus medius began to fire prior to toe-off and was active throughout swing phase. This abnormal muscle activity explained the circumduction of the limb in swing phase. The phasic prolongation of the gluteus maximus in stance phase was part of the compensatory mechanism for stability of the limb in stance phase.

Force plate measurements of the right lower extremity revealed impaired loading, diminished forward shear and absent aft shear,

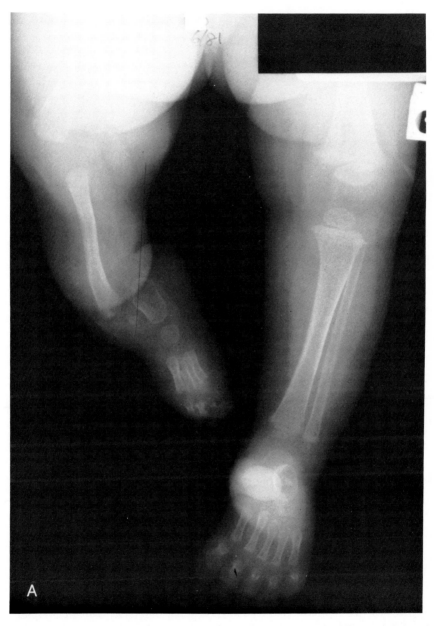

Figure 7.3. (A) Patient R.O.: congenital terminal right tibial hemimelia and accessory toe on the medial dorsal aspect of the left foot. X-ray of lower extremities at age 9 months.

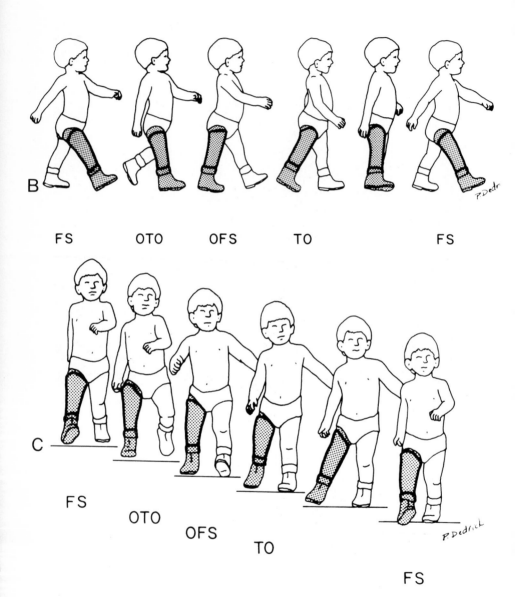

Figure 7.3. (B and C) Patient R.O. Tracings of film from right side (B) and front (C) camera with patient wearing nonarticulated lower extremity prosthesis. (See Fig. 7.1 for abbreviations.)

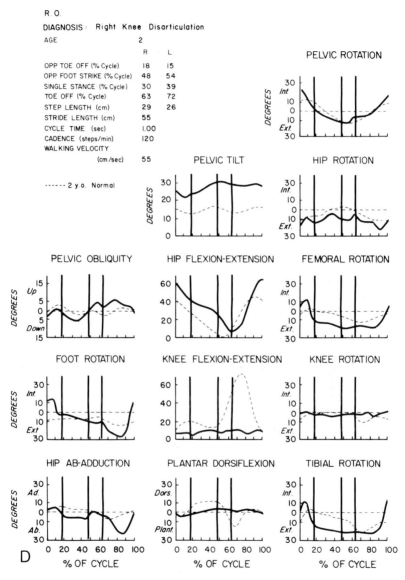

R.O.

DIAGNOSIS : Right Knee Disarticulation

AGE 2

	R	L
OPP TOE OFF (% Cycle)	18	15
OPP FOOT STRIKE (% Cycle)	48	54
SINGLE STANCE (% Cycle)	30	39
TOE OFF (% Cycle)	63	72
STEP LENGTH (cm)	29	26
STRIDE LENGTH (cm)	55	
CYCLE TIME (sec)	1.00	
CADENCE (steps/min)	120	
WALKING VELOCITY (cm/sec)	55	

------ 2 y.o. Normal

Figure 7.3. (*D*) Patient R.O. Linear measurements and joint angle rotations. Joint angle rotations are compared with values for normal 2-year-old subjects.

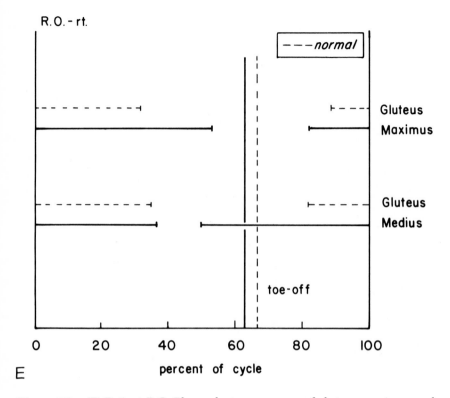

Figure 7.3.   (*E*) Patient R.O. Phase electromyograms of gluteus maximus and gluteus medius compared with normal 2-year-old subjects.

calcaneal concentration of center of pressure and increased lateral shear (Fig. 7.3F).

Force plate measurements of the left lower extremity showed exaggerated loading, increased forward shear, increased lateral shear, and an abnormal pattern of center of pressure progression with concentration of center of pressure in the hind foot and mid-foot. There was no apparent explanation for this abnormal center of pressure progression on the contralateral side.

The nonarticulated above-knee prosthesis clearly imposed demands of additional energy which the child at this age has in abundance. The asymmetrical force plate measurements and the marked compensatory movements required by the right stiff knee suggest the likelihood of a high energy output in walking. A prosthesis with the knee joint will be applied when the child is approximately 3½ or 4 years old, when mature walking has been achieved, and he is able to adapt to a more complex prosthesis.

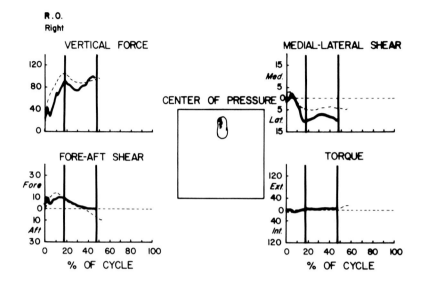

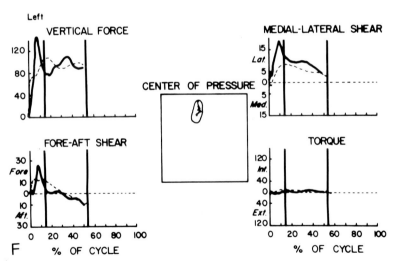

Figure 7.3. (F) Patient R.O. Force plate measurements, right and left lower extremities, with normal 2-year-old subjects for comparison.

References

1. Aitken GT: The childhood amputee—an overview. *Orthop Clin North Am* 3:447–472, 1972.
2. Brown FW: Construction of a knee joint in congenital total absence of the tibia (paraxial hemimelia tibia). A preliminary report. *J Bone Joint Surg* 47A:695–704, 1965.

3. Condie DN: Ankle foot mechanisms. In Murdoch G: *Prosthetic and Orthotic Practice*. London, Edward Arnold, 1970, pp 89–103.
4. Davidson WH, Bohne WHO: The Syme amputation in children. *J Bone Joint Surg* 57A:905–908, 1975.
5. Foort J: The Canadian type Syme prosthesis. Lower Extremity Research Project. Institute of Engineering Research, University of California at Berkeley. Report to the Prosthetic Research Board, National Research Council, Series 11, Issue 30, December 1956.
6. Frantz CH, O'Rahilly R: Congenital skeletal limb deficiencies. *J Bone Joint Surg* 43A:1202–1220, 1961.
7. Hueter C: Anatomische Studien an den Extremitätengelenken Neugeborener und Erwachsener. *Arch Pathol Anat* 25:527–599, 1962.
8. Lambert CN: Amputation surgery on the child. *Orthop Clin North Am* 3:473–482, 1972.
9. Von Soal G: Epiphyseodesis combined with amputation. *J Bone Joint Surg* 21:442–443, 1939.
10. Wilson B: Prostheses for Syme amputation. *Artif Limbs* 6:56–74, 1961.

CHAPTER 8

Nonprogressive Spinal Cord and Peripheral Nerve Disorders

INTRODUCTION

A number of diverse problems are discussed in this chapter, and the cases presented have a single common denominator: the absence of progression of the neurologic disorder being reviewed. The first three examples deal with motor problems due to lower motor neuron or peripheral nerve disorders. In the last case, motor paresis was superimposed on spasticity secondary to prematurity.

The control system is usually intact in the subjects with lower motor neuron disease. This means that muscles which function well can be used to perform some of the functions of the paralyzed muscles. An example of this kind of substitution is steppage gait—increased hip and knee flexion to clear the foot in swing phase when the muscles of the anterior compartment are paralyzed. An instance of this functional substitution is noted in this chapter. Previous electromyographic studies have shown gluteus maximus and hamstring phase prolongation in patients with quadriceps weakness from poliomyelitis (7). Numerous phase alterations were evident in both the transplanted and nontransplanted muscles.

Why include poliomyelitis when immunization has virtually eliminated this disease in many parts of the world? In the San Diego community, there has been a recent influx of patients who had incurred the disease in Southeast Asia, and for years patients who contracted the disease in Mexico, Central America or South America have come to Children's Hospital in San Diego. Many of these patients need surgery or bracing because of residual paralysis from poliomyelitis. Most of the literature on poliomyelitis rehabilitation antedates the clinical application of motion analysis, and there is still much to be learned. Careful motion analysis studies prior to treatment facilitate rational treatment planning, and follow-up studies allow assessment of treatment outcome.

POLIOMYELITIS

Patient A.E. contracted poliomyelitis at 4 years of age and was left with severe weakness of the right lower extremity. Tendoachilles lengthening and peroneus brevis transfers to the mid-foot were performed at 9 years of age. Long-leg bracing was necessary following surgery, and the patient was brace-dependent when gait study was

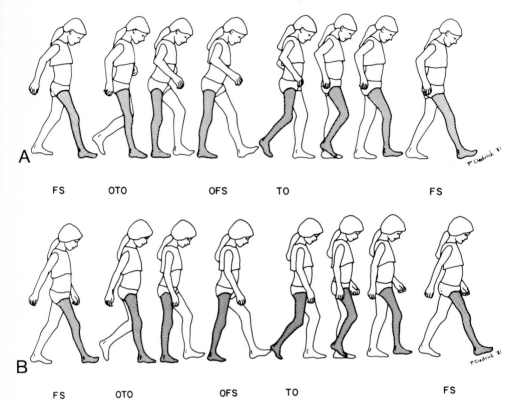

FS   OTO   OFS   TO   FS

FS   OTO   OFS   TO   FS

Figure 8.1. (A and B) Patient A.E.: Post-poliomyelitis, instability of right lower extremity. (A) Film tracings from right side camera. (B) Six months following total transfer of semitendinosus and semimembranosus to reinforce knee extension. (FS = foot-strike, OTO = opposite toe-off, OFS = opposite foot-strike, and TO = toe-off.)

done at 10 years. She could walk only a short distance without the support of a long-leg brace with knee locked.

The right limb was atrophied and short 4.4 cm by scanogram measurement. Muscle strength: hip flexors, 4; adductors, 4; gluteus maximus, 5; gluteus medius, 3; quadriceps, 1; hamstrings, 4; ankle plantar flexors, −4.

Gait Assessment

Tracings of one walk cycle from the right side camera (Fig. 8.1A) showed forward trunk lean throughout single-limb support (OTO to OFS), and diminished hip extension (OFS). Left step length was shorter than the right. (See OFS and FS.)

Film tracings from the front camera showed a gluteus medius lurch (Fig. 8.1C). Cadence and velocity were low (94 steps per minute and

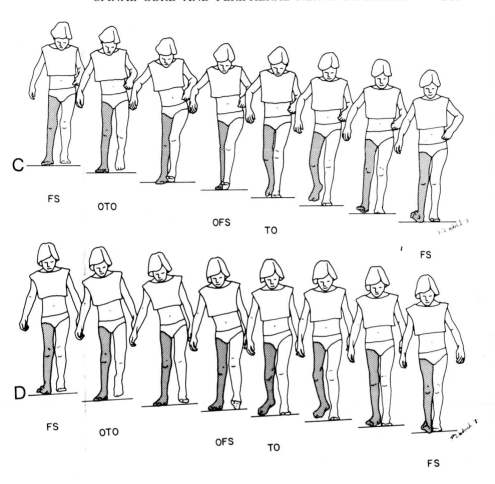

Figure 8.1. (*C* and *D*) Patient A.E. (*C*) Film tracings from front camera. (*D*) Six months following total transfer of semitendinosus and semimembranosus to reinforce knee extension.

45 cm per second) (Fig. 8.1E). Step lengths were asymmetrical—right, 31 cm, and left, 26 cm. The duration of single stance was 21% on the right and 39% on the left. The short single stance on the right was due to limb instability.

Excessive anterior pelvic tilt was present during stance phase (Fig. 8.1E). The hip remained in flexion through stance phase (Fig. 8.1F). The knee flexed slightly at foot-strike, extended almost to neutral at the beginning of single-limb support, but then gradually flexed to 35° at the end of stance (Fig. 8.1F). The foot was plantar-flexed at foot-

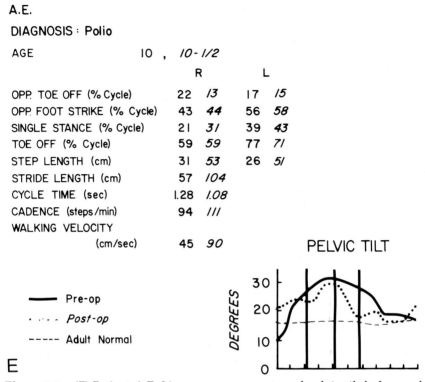

A.E.

DIAGNOSIS : Polio

AGE   10 , *10 - 1/2*

	R		L	
OPP. TOE OFF (% Cycle)	22	*13*	17	*15*
OPP. FOOT STRIKE (% Cycle)	43	*44*	56	*58*
SINGLE STANCE (% Cycle)	21	*31*	39	*43*
TOE OFF (% Cycle)	59	*59*	77	*71*
STEP LENGTH (cm)	31	*53*	26	*51*
STRIDE LENGTH (cm)	57	*104*		
CYCLE TIME (sec)	1.28	*1.08*		
CADENCE (steps/min)	94	*111*		
WALKING VELOCITY (cm/sec)	45	*90*		

——— Pre-op

· ··· · *Post-op*

– – – – Adult Normal

PELVIC TILT

E

Figure 8.1. (E) Patient A.E. Linear measurements and pelvic tilt before and after surgery with adult normal values for comparison of pelvic tilt.

strike and showed progressive dorsiflexion until opposite foot-strike (calcaneal pattern) (Fig. 8.1F).

Floor reaction measurements for the right lower extremity (Fig. 8.1G) demonstrated impaired loading and impaired push-off. Fore and aft shear were diminished; lateral shear was absent; and excessive internal torque occurred throughout stance.

Assessment of this gait indicated that right lower extremity instability prevented stable load bearing. Gait measurements when correlated with clinical data showed that inability to control knee flexion was the primary deficit. Hamstring transfer to the patella was selected from the options available for treatment. Weakness of the triceps surae and quadriceps required an innovative approach—total transfer of two medial hamstrings to reinforce knee extension. The proximal origins of the semitendinosus and semimembranosus were removed from the ischial tuberosity and transferred to the femur. The muscle insertions were redirected anteriorly to insert into the patella. The rationale of this approach related to maintenance of tension in the two-joint

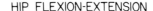

HIP FLEXION-EXTENSION

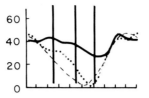

KNEE FLEXION-EXTENSION

PLANTAR DORSIFLEXION

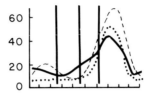

30
Dors.
10
0
10
Plant.
30

0 20 40 60 80 100

F   % OF CYCLE

A.E.

Right

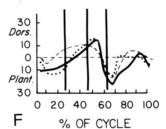

VERTICAL FORCE

120
80
40
0

CENTER OF PRESSURE

MEDIAL-LATERAL SHEAR

15
Med.
5
0
5
Lat.
15

FORE-AFT SHEAR

30
Fore
10
0
10
Aft
30

0 20 40 60 80 100

G   % OF CYCLE

—— Pre-op
..... Post-op

TORQUE

120
Ext.
40
0
40
Int.
120

0 20 40 60 80 100

% OF CYCLE

Figure 8.1. (F and G) Patient A.E. Sagittal plane hip, knee and ankle movements before and after surgery (F), and force plate measurements, right lower extremity, before and after surgery (G), with adult normal values for comparison.

muscles throughout the required range of function (2–5, 7). When only the distal hamstring tendons are transferred anteriorly to the patella, effective tension is lost as the hip extends (7). In this patient, weakness of the calf group necessitated a longer time of action to cover both load acceptance when the hip was flexed and resistance to knee flexion through the rest of the stance when the hip was extended. Conversion of the semitendinosus and semimembranosus muscles to a one-joint muscle eliminated this hindrance to effective function. This muscle transfer should be considered only when the gluteus maximus is strong. The hamstring muscles have important hip extension function which is lost when the muscle origins are removed from the ischial tuberosity.

After the operative procedure, the patient gained sufficient stability in the limb to discard her brace. She was seen regularly in follow-up examinations for 6 years and remained a community ambulator, requiring no bracing. Leg length inequality was corrected by left distal femoral and proximal tibial epiphyseodesis.

Film tracings from the side camera 6 months postoperatively showed improvement in step length, loss of forward trunk lean, and less hip flexion during single-limb support (Fig. 8.1B). Postoperative film tracings from the front camera showed continuation of the gluteus medius lurch (Fig. 8.1D and C). However, some improvement in arm alignment was noted, particularly in the left arm. This was attributed to better stability during single-limb stance. The changes in cadence, velocity and step length were striking (Fig. 8.1E). Duration of single stance increased from 21 to 31 on the right. Walking velocity doubled, increasing from 45 to 90. Cadence increased from 94 to 111 steps per minute. Step length increased on the right from 31 to 53 cm (71%), and on the left from 26 to 51 cm (96%). These measurements clearly imply that the increase in walking velocity was largely due to the tremendous increase in step length.

The changes in motion were equally dramatic. The primary change was better alignment at the hip, with restoration of normal hip extension in stance phase (Fig. 8.1F). The knee remained fully extended in stance phase. Had the hamstring transfers been sufficiently strong to restore full stability to the knee in walking, the knee flexion wave would have been restored, and single stance on the right would have more closely approached a normal value. Knee extension strength at the time of the 6-month follow-up was 3−, comparing with 1 before transfer. The postoperative right limb vertical force, initial loading, and push-off phases were much improved, and lateral shear increased (Fig. 8.1G). These changes resulted from increased limb stability.

Gait analysis was valuable in planning treatment for this patient, and indispensable in evaluating the outcome.

GUILLAIN-BARRÉ SYNDROME

Patient C.M. became quadriplegic following symptoms of Guillain-Barré's syndrome at age 14. Over a 19-month period, muscle strength gradually returned to all muscle groups except those below the knees. At the time of the gait study, walking was difficult without ankle support, but with bilateral polypropylene ankle-foot orthoses, the patient could walk fairly well.

No contractures were present. Examination of motor power revealed minor weakness of hip and thigh muscles, but major paralysis was present below the knees.

Muscle strength:

	Right	Left
Hip flexors	4+	4+
Gluteus maximus	4+	4+
Gluteus medius	4+	4+
Quadriceps femoris	4+	4+
Hamstrings	4	4
Triceps surae	2	2
Toe extensors	0	0
Tibialis anterior	0	1
Peroneals	0	0

Gait analysis was done to compare walking with and without polypropylene ankle-foot orthoses.

Tracings of film from the right side camera without orthoses (Fig. 8.2A) showed flat foot-strike, extended knee during single-limb stance, drop foot and exaggerated hip flexion in early swing phase. This exaggeration of hip flexion, a compensatory movement for foot drop, is commonly referred to as steppage gait. Film tracings from the right camera with the patient wearing orthoses (Fig. 8.2B) exhibited the following gait improvements: restoration of heel-strike, increased step length, and reduction of hyperflexion in swing phase. Extension of the knee in stance phase persisted.

Film tracings from the front camera of walk cycle without orthoses (Fig. 8.2C) showed abnormally wide ankle spread. Film tracings from the front camera with the patient wearing orthoses demonstrated diminished ankle spread (Fig. 8.2D). Significant improvement in walking velocity, cadence, and stride length occurred when orthoses were worn (Fig. 8.2E). Stride length increased from 73 to 106 cm; cadence, 85 to 101 steps per minute; and walking velocity from 52 to 89 cm per second. Pelvic rotation was restored to normal with the orthoses which also improved anterior pelvic tilt, corrected hyperflexion of the hip in swing phase, and improved ankle motion.

The use of orthoses also improved floor reaction measurements for both lower extremities. Initial loading, forward shear, and lateral shear

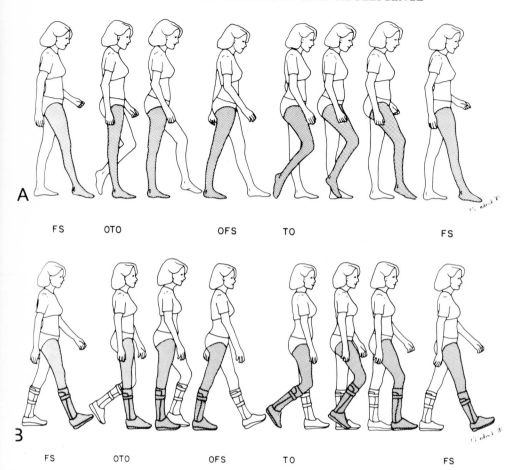

A

FS   OTO   OFS   TO   FS

B

FS   OTO   OFS   TO   FS

Figure 8.2. (A and B) Patient C.M.: Guillain-Barré's disease. Tracings of film from right side camera (A) and with bilateral ankle-foot orthoses (B). (See Fig. 8.1 for abbreviations.)

increased. The calcaneal pattern of center of pressure progression improved slightly (8) (Fig. 8.2F).

To summarize the findings, this patient with Guillain-Barré's syndrome benefited markedly from wearing bilateral ankle-foot orthoses. Drop foot was well controlled, but calcaneal weakness still dominated the pattern and explained the relatively slow gait (8). The patient's walking velocity and stability might be improved by arthrodesis of the ankle joints. However, she did not find her present disability sufficient to consider surgical treatment. She also believed that she was still recovering strength. The plan is to continue observation and orthotic management.

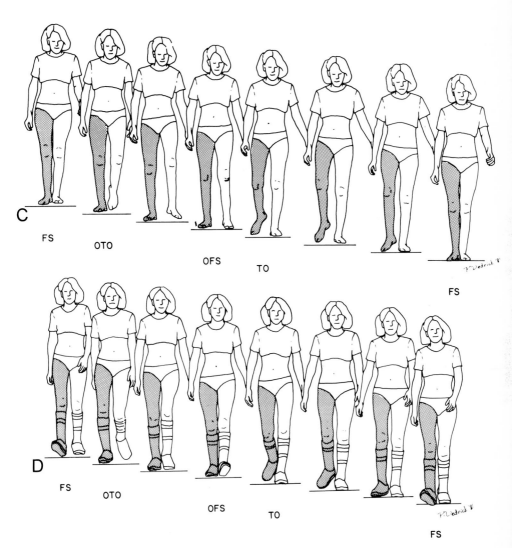

Figure 8.2. (C and D) Patient C.M. Tracings of film from front camera (C) and with bilateral ankle-foot orthoses (D).

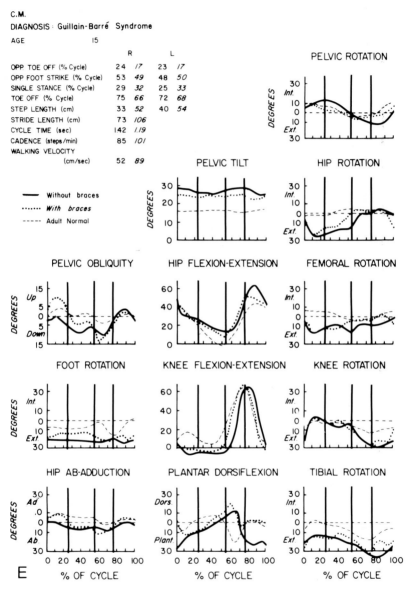

Figure 8.2.   (E) Patient C.M. Linear measurements and joint angle measurements with and without braces. Adult normal angles are given for comparison.

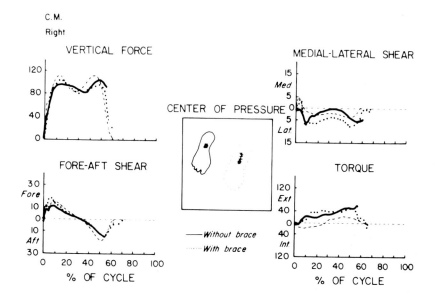

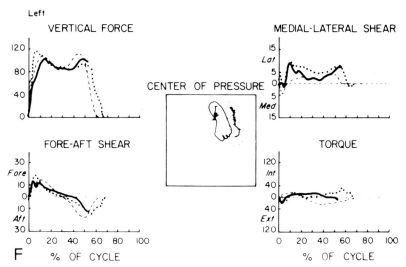

Figure 8.2. (F) Patient C.M. Floor reaction forces for right and left lower extremities with and without braces. Adult normal force plate values are given for comparison (*broken lines*).

PERIPHERAL NERVE INJURY

Patient J.S. developed drop foot following injection into the left buttock at age 2 years. Past medical history was uneventful. The

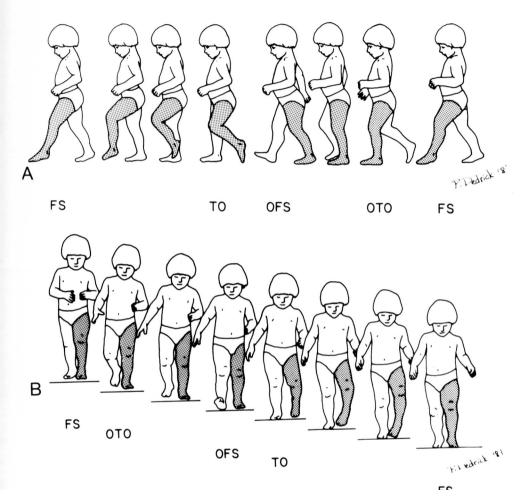

Figure 8.3. (A and B) Patient J.S.: paralytic foot drop following injection into left buttock. Tracings of film from left (A) and front (B) camera. (See Fig. 8.1 for abbreviations.)

muscles of the anterior and lateral compartments were completely paralyzed, except for a trace of voluntary muscle activity in the peroneus longus and brevis. Electromyographic studies demonstrated peroneal nerve involvement, including the short head of the biceps femoris. The pediatric neurologist who conducted the electromyographic study concluded that the findings were consistent with a sciatic nerve injury secondary to injection into the buttock. A polypropylene ankle-foot orthosis was prescribed by the orthopaedist and was being used regularly at the time of the gait study. Walking was evaluated without orthosis 3 months after the onset of paralysis.

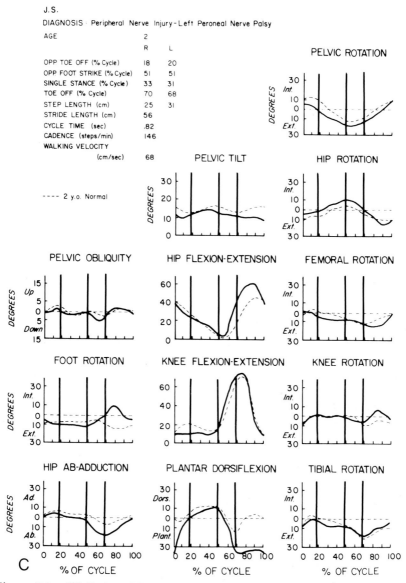

J.S.

DIAGNOSIS : Peripheral Nerve Injury-Left Peroneal Nerve Palsy

		R	L
AGE		2	
OPP TOE OFF (% Cycle)		18	20
OPP FOOT STRIKE (% Cycle)		51	51
SINGLE STANCE (% Cycle)		33	31
TOE OFF (% Cycle)		70	68
STEP LENGTH (cm)		25	31
STRIDE LENGTH (cm)		56	
CYCLE TIME (sec)		.82	
CADENCE (steps/min)		146	
WALKING VELOCITY (cm/sec)		68	

---- 2 y.o. Normal

Figure 8.3. (C) Patient J.S. Linear measurements and joint angle rotations, shown with values for normal 2-year-old subjects for comparison.

Results of the study are shown to outline characteristic features of paralytic foot drop.

Film tracings from the side camera (Fig. 8.3A) showed flat foot-strike, followed by normal ankle dorsiflexion in stance phase and 30° equinus in swing phase. Clearance of the foot was accomplished by exaggerated hip flexion in swing phase. The other significant movement abnormality was internal rotation of the foot in swing phase, due to the effects of gravity unopposed by muscle action (Fig. 8.3, *B* and *C*).

The patient's walking velocity was slow as compared with the average for a 2-year-old child (Fig. 8.3*C*). Step lengths were asymmetrical, with the right step 25 cm, and the left, 31 cm. The duration of single stance was reduced on the right.

The gait abnormalities displayed in this patient are typical of paralytic foot drop, with total paralysis of the anterior and lateral compartment muscles (9). Paralytic foot drop is primarily a swing phase problem, and accordingly this child showed little difficulty in stance phase. Paralytic foot drop produces much less impairment in locomotion than paralysis of the triceps surae (8, 9). The patient was easily managed with a polypropylene ankle-foot orthosis, and muscle function gradually returned to normal. A gait study, not shown, repeated 1 year and 5 months after the injection showed entirely symmetrical lower extremity movements, and the orthosis had been discarded.

SPINAL CORD INJURY

Patient R.A. presented with an unusual history and a complex motion disorder. He was the product of premature delivery and a diagnosis of cerebral palsy was made in the first year of life. At 15 months of age, he fell, sustaining a cervical injury with total quadriplegia. He was treated by skeletal traction, utilizing skull tongs, and partial recovery of function resulted. Additional surgery to stabilize the spine was considered, but apparently rejected as being too dangerous. X-rays taken at age 7 revealed an ununited fracture of the neural arch of C-3 and multiple anomalies of the upper cervical spine, including fusion of the body of C-2 to the cranium (Fig. 8.4, *A* and *B*). The patient then underwent an occipital to C-2 posterior fusion with halo immobilization. This surgery restored cervical stability and provided protection to the spinal cord (Fig. 8.4*C*). Both spasticity and weakness were noted, and ambulatory function was restricted to household level. Increased muscle tone in the right upper and lower extremities and muscle contractures were present: hip extension, $-30/-30$; knee extension, $-15/-5$; ankle dorsiflexion, $-10/0$. The child walked with a crablike gait with some constant pelvic rotation, restricted right step length, and restricted right hip extension.

Film tracings from the right side camera (Fig. 8.4*D*) showed asymmetric gait with short step length and poorly coordinated arm and leg movements. Film tracings from the front camera showed malrotation of the pelvis, adduction and internal rotation of the right lower extremity, and poorly coordinated arm movements (Fig. 8.4*F*). Electromyog-

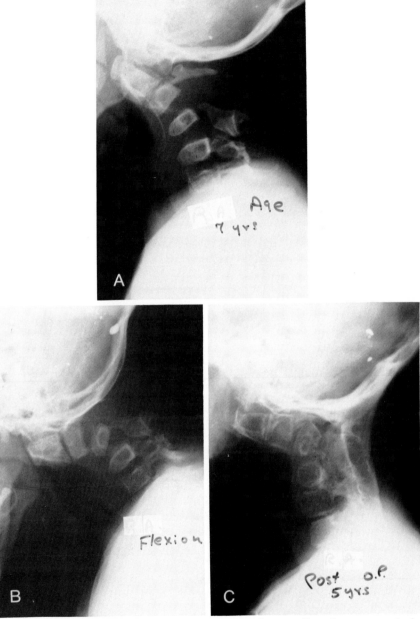

Figure 8.4. (A–C) Patient R.A., age 7: congenital anomalies of upper cervical spine, spinal instability, and spinal cord injury. Preoperative x-ray (A) and film showing spinal instability in flexion (B). (C) X-ray 5 years following occipital cervical fusion.

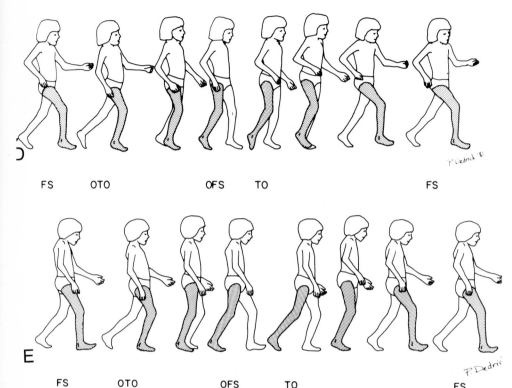

FS   OTO   OFS   TO   FS

FS   OTO   OFS   TO   FS

Figure 8.4.   (D and E) Patient R.A. Tracings from right side camera, preoperative (D) and postoperative (E). (See Fig. 8.1 for abbreviations.)

raphy revealed marked overactivity in the right iliacus muscle and adductor longus (Fig. 8.4H). Force plate measurements showed increased initial loading in both limbs and an equinus pattern of center of pressure in both limbs (Fig. 8.4I). Walking velocity was restricted, and step lengths were asymmetrical, with the right shorter than the left (Fig. 8.4J). On the basis of the measured movement abnormalities (Fig. 8.4J) and the abnormal muscle activity (8.4H), the treatment selected included bilateral posterior adductor transfers, right iliopsoas lengthening, and right posterior tibialis lengthening. Postoperative film tracings from the side camera 1 year and 3 months following surgery show increase in step length, improvement in right hip extension, and better coordinated hand movements (Fig. 8.4E). Film tracings from the front camera demonstrate better alignment of the right lower extremity and better coordinated hand and arm movements (Fig. 8.4G).

Cadence dropped while velocity increased, and stride length advanced from 71 to 84 cm (Fig. 8.4J). Step lengths were more symmet-

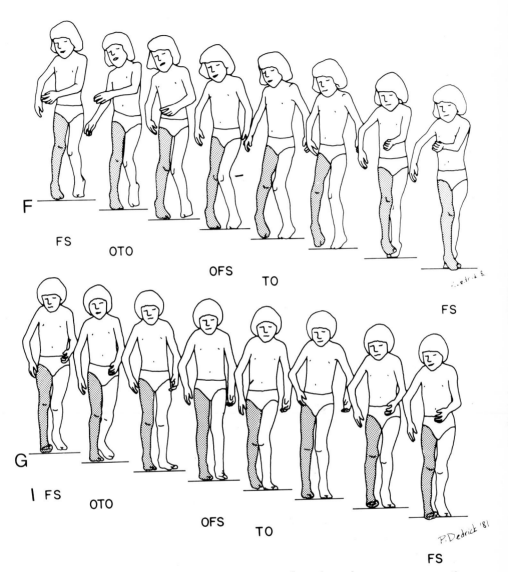

Figure 8.4. (F and G) Patient R.A. Tracings from frontal camera, preoperative (F) and postoperative (G).

rical after surgery. Bilateral polypropylene ankle-foot orthoses were utilized, and an additional study (not shown) done on the same day with orthoses showed further improvement in walking velocity and step length. With the orthoses, velocity increased to 96 cm per second, representing a 33% increase as compared with preoperative status.

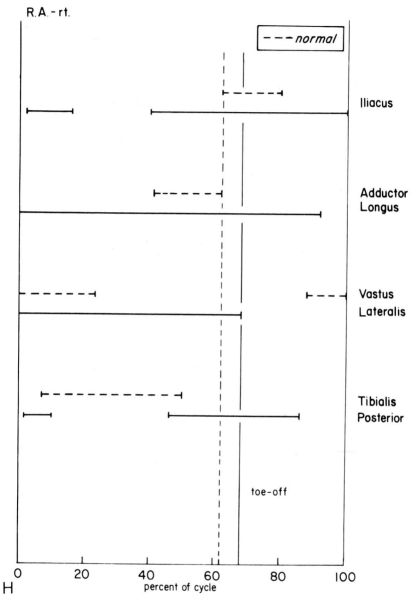

Figure 8.4. (*H*) Patient R.A. Preoperative electromyograms with adult normal values for comparison.

Little change occurred in the force plate measurements, except for center of pressure distribution which indicated slight improvement in both feet (Fig. 8.4*I*).

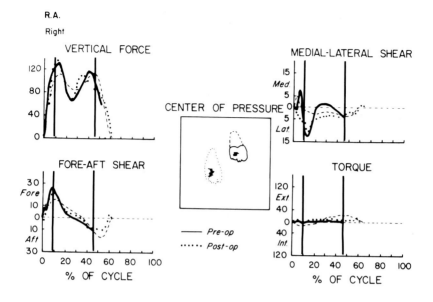

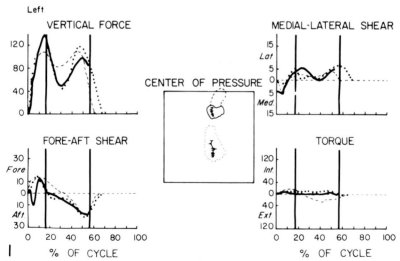

Figure 8.4. (*I*) Patient R.A. Force plate measurements pre- and postoperatively with adult normal values (*broken lines*) for comparison.

The clinical changes in this child following surgery were significant. His functional level advanced from household to community ambulation.

126   GAIT DISORDERS IN CHILDHOOD AND ADOLESCENCE

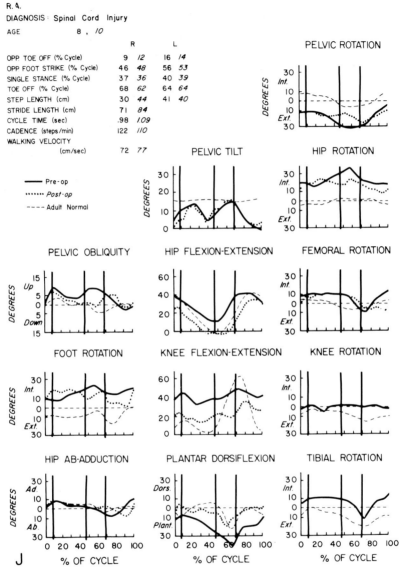

Figure 8.4. (*J*) Patient R.A. Linear measurements and joint angle rotation before and after surgery with adult normal values for comparison.

References

1. Asbury AK, Arnason BG, Adams RD: The inflammatory lesion in idiopathic polyneuritis. *Medicine* 48:173–215, 1969.
2. Brunnstrom S: Knee region: discussion of function of muscles of knee. In *Clinical Kinesiology*, Ed. 3. Philadelphia, F.A. Davis, 1972, Chap 6, pp 189–191.
3. MacConaill MA, Basmajian JV: Hip, thigh and leg. In *Muscles and Movements: A*

Basis for Human Kinesiology, Ed. 2. Huntington, N.Y., Robert E. Krieger, 1977, Chap 13, pp 308–309.
4. Markee JE, Logue JT, Williams M, et al: Two-joint muscles of the thigh. *J Bone Joint Surg* 37A:125–142, 1955.
5. O'Connell AL, Gardner EB: Mechanics of muscle action. In *Understanding the Scientific Bases of Human Movement*. Baltimore, Williams & Wilkins, 1972, Chap 2, p 38.
6. Silfverskiöld N: Reduction of the uncrossed two-joint muscles of the leg to one-joint muscles in spastic conditions. *Acta Chir Scand* 56:315–330, 1923–24.
7. Sutherland DH, Bost FC, Schottstaedt ER: Electromyographic study of transplanted muscles about the knee in poliomyelitis patients. *J Bone Joint Surg* 42A:919–939, 1960.
8. Sutherland DH, Cooper L, Daniel D: The role of the ankle plantar flexors in normal walking. *J Bone Joint Surg* 62A:354–363, 1980.
9. Sutherland DH, Baumann JU: Correction of foot drop by external orthoses. In Black J, Dumbleton JH: *Clinical Biomechanics: A Case History Approach*. New York, Churchill Livingstone, 1981, Chap 14, pp 307–316.

CHAPTER 9

Disorders of Motor Control

NONPROGRESSIVE DISORDER: CEREBRAL PALSY

Cerebral palsy is defined as "the disorder to movement and posture due to defect or lesion of the immature brain" (1). This definition stresses the importance of perceiving and analyzing movement in cerebral palsy. The defect lies in the brain, but recognizing the disorder, identifying the subtypes, and attempting to plan rational treatment all depend wholly upon demonstrating specific movement abnormalities. The control system in the brain is directly at fault, and the muscles are indirectly involved through improper activation signals. Patients with cerebral palsy, unlike those who have lower motor neuron disorders, often lack well-defined compensatory movements, and the sequence of activation of various muscles is frequently abnormal. Prolonged electromyographic activity, patterning (simultaneous activity in several muscle groups), and concurrent activity of both agonist and antagonist muscles can result from malfunction of the control system. In contrast with muscular dystrophy, the movement disorder in cerebral palsy is usually asymmetrical.

Three of the most common clinical presentations in cerebral palsy are spastic hemiplegia, spastic diplegia, and spastic quadriplegia. These clinical designations allow for general groupings of patients. However, many qualitative and quantitative differences are present even in patients who seem to fit into clinical categories. Hemiplegia refers to those with upper and lower extremity involvement on the same side. Diplegia indicates involvement of both lower extremities. Quadriplegic subjects have involvement of the trunk and all four extremities. Spasticity is characterized by increased stretch reflexes and clonus, and a positive Babinski and Hoffmann test. Spasticity in cerebral palsy is due to a pyramidal tract disorder.

Extrapyramidal types of cerebral palsy display a number of more complex movement abnormalities (2). Athetosis is characterized by intermittent assumption of abnormal postural attitudes. Athetoid movements tend to affect the peripheral musculature of the limbs and face and are more pronounced distally than proximally in the extremities. Choreoathetoid movements are similar, but are more abrupt, brief and jerky. Dystonic movements involve larger portions of the body, i.e. an entire extremity or the trunk. Ballismus is rare and involves large-scale, violent tossing or flinging motion. Regular alternating movements signify tremor. The term "rigidity" is used when resistance to passive movements occurs throughout the entire range of motion. Physical and occupational therapy, surgery, and orthotics all have important roles in the management of the motor-skeletal aspects of cerebral palsy. These patients have multiple needs, depending upon the extent and location of the brain defect. Some require special education, counseling, speech therapy, eye surgery, communication and mobility aids.

The examples that follow are three patients with the pyramidal tract type of cerebral palsy—the most common manifestation. They differ sharply in the quantity of involvement progressing from the least (hemiplegia) to the greatest (quadriplegia). From the description, it may seem that walking in cerebral palsy is chaotic and totally lacking in pattern. On the contrary, examination of multiple cycles in one subject usually points up a remarkable regularity in cycle repetition.

Hemiplegia

Patient J.W. was noted to have right hemiparesis in the first year of life. His developmental milestones were mildly delayed. Treatment consisted of regular physical and occupational therapy. At 4 years of age, right heel cord lengthening was performed. The equinus contracture recurred and he was referred for gait analysis at the age of 9.

Examination revealed impairment of selective control of the right upper extremity. Deep tendon reflexes in the right arm and leg were hyperactive, and there was a positive Babinski test on the right. There were no muscle contractures of the right hip or knee. The triceps surae was contracted, limiting passive dorsiflexion to $-10°$ with the knee flexed, and $-20°$ with the knee extended. Mild inversion of the foot and prominence of the posterior tibial tendon behind the medial malleolus were noted. Characteristic features of hemiplegia are seen in tracings of film from the right side camera (Fig. 9.1A). At the time of foot strike, the right ankle was in equinus and toe contact was made before heel contact. Ankle equinus continued throughout stance phase and persisted in swing phase. The right elbow was flexed during single-limb support. Film from the front camera showed arm posturing (elbow and wrist flexed, shoulder abducted). Ankle varus was present during initial double support and swing phase (Fig. 9.1B). Abnormal joint movements noted from the side were increased anterior pelvic tilt, internal rotation of the foot, increased external rotation of the pelvis in stance phase, increased hip adduction in stance phase, and marked equinus of the ankle throughout the gait cycle (Fig. 9.1C). The tibialis posterior and soleus muscles began activity prematurely in late swing phase. The tibialis anterior showed relatively normal phasic activity.

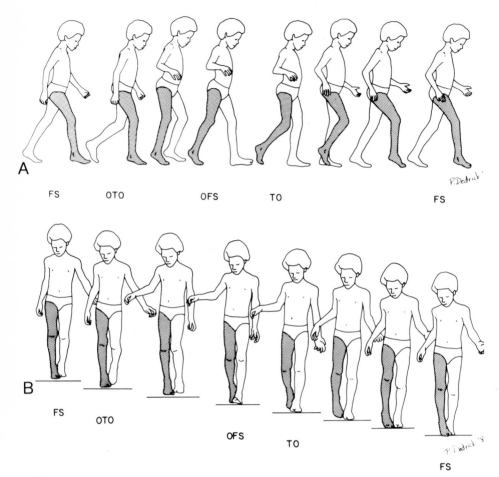

Figure 9.1.   (A and B) Patient J.W., age 9 years: right hemiplegia. Preoperative tracings from side (A) and front (B) camera. (FS = foot-strike, OTO = opposite toe-off, OFS = opposite foot-strike, TO = toe-off.)

Stance phase activity of the lateral hamstrings, vastus medialis, and vastus lateralis was prolonged (Fig. 9.1D).

Perry and Hoffer (5) recommended that muscle transfers in patients with cerebral palsy be limited to muscles which show electromyographic activity in the desired phase. For example, the posterior tibialis muscle should not be used for transfer unless it functions primarily in swing phase. Based on this criterion, posterior tibial tendon transfer in patient J.W. would not be appropriate. The author recommended

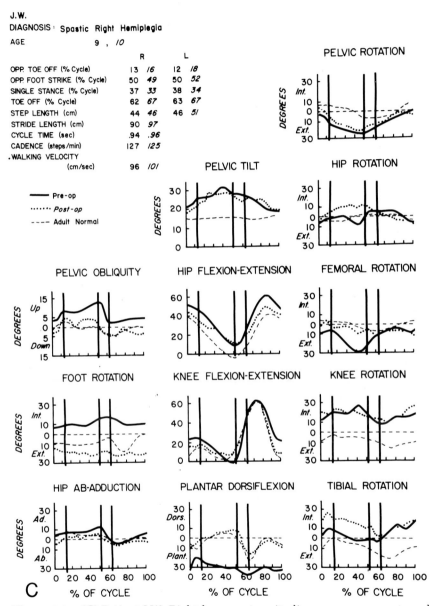

Figure 9.1.   (C) Patient J.W. Right lower extremity linear measurements and joint angles pre- and postoperatively, with comparison of adult normal values.

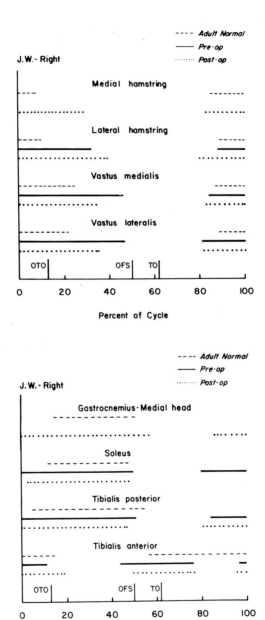

Figure 9.1. (*D*) Patient J.W. Pre- and postoperative phase electromyograms with adult normal values for comparison.

lengthening of the tendoachilles and the tibialis posterior, but the referring surgeon transferred the tibialis posterior through the interosseous space to the dorsum of the foot and lengthened the tendoachilles.

ASSESSMENT

The early result is shown in tracings of film from the right side camera 12 months following surgery (Fig. 9.1E). Gait improvements included: restoration of heel-strike, correction of equinus, and im-

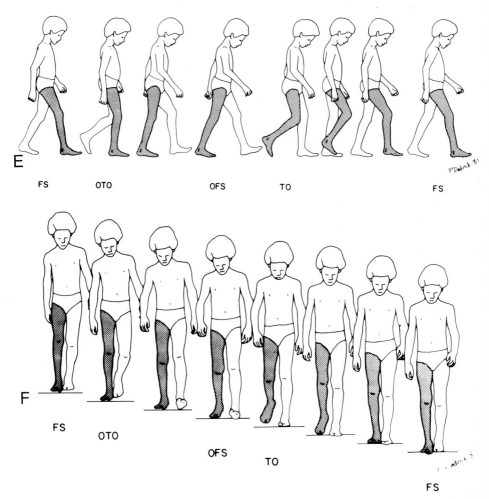

E

FS   OTO   OFS   TO   FS

F

FS   OTO

                              OFS   TO

                                                                   FS

Figure 9.1. (E and F) Patient J.W. Film tracings 1 year after tendoachilles lengthening and posterior tibial transfer through the interosseous space to dorsum of the foot, side (E) and front (F) camera.

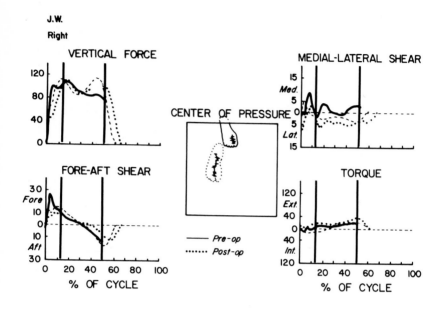

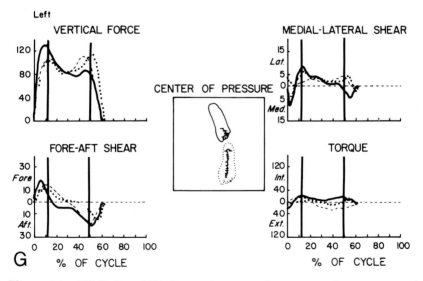

Figure 9.1. (G) Patient J.W. Force plate recording pre- and postoperatively with adult normal values for comparison.

provement in arm positioning. Tracings of film from the front camera showed slight valgus of the right foot and reduction of right shoulder abduction (Fig. 9.1F). Stride length was increased, cadence dropped slightly, and walking velocity increased minimally (Fig. 9.1C). Ankle motion became normal, exaggerated hip flexion in swing phase was corrected, and hip movement in the coronal plane (hip adduction/abduction) became more normal. Electromyographic activity in the tibialis posterior was unchanged (Fig. 9.1D). The postoperative floor reaction measurements showed considerable improvement (Fig. 9.1G). On the sound limb, rapid and excessive loading, early shear, and concentration of the center of pressure in the forefoot were present before surgery and absent in the postoperative study. The preoperative measurements in the right lower extremity showed rapid loading, increased forward shear, absent lateral shear, and concentration of pressure in the forefoot. Postoperatively, all of the measurements were nearly normal.

DISCUSSION

Improvement in swing phase dorsiflexion must be attributed to the elimination of equinus contracture, because the tibialis posterior which was transferred to the dorsum of the foot was inactive during early and mid-swing. The improvement in the arm movements is attributed to removal of the need for compensation. Apparently, the compensatory arm posturing was no longer required after the improvement of ankle and foot stability. By objective criteria, this treatment was successful. However, a note of caution must be introduced. Gait study (not shown) was repeated 2 years after the initial surgery, revealing some increase in the valgus alignment of the foot. On this most recent study, the foot was in 25° external rotation through the gait cycle. This change indicates that there has been some alteration of the mediolateral balance of the foot secondary to loss of the medial stabilizing effect of the tibialis posterior. The patient remains functionally excellent, but additional follow-up will be required to determine if valgus increases, necessitating further operative treatment.

Spastic Diplegia

Patient D.M., a 16-year-old boy, was a product of premature birth and breech delivery. He was cyanotic at birth and was cared for in an infant intensive care unit for 3 months. Developmental milestones were delayed. He talked at 2 years of age, but did not walk independently until shortly after surgical lengthenings of the right and left tendoachilles and lengthening of the right medial hamstring tendons.

At the age of 14, the patient could walk, run, and play basketball, but knee flexion was excessive and he complained of intermittent knee pain. Coordination of the lower extremities was impaired. There were bilateral hip flexion contractures of 20°, right knee flexion contracture of 30°, and left knee flexion contracture of 10°. The right ankle could be dorsiflexed to neutral and the left ankle could be brought to +10°. X-rays of the knees confirmed the presence of patellae altae. X-rays of the hips showed good femoral head coverage and no subluxation.

Tracings from the left side camera film showed excessive knee flexion and exaggerated ankle dorsiflexion during single limb support (Fig. 9.2A). Body weight and inertia exerted powerful flexion torque on the knee, necessitating strong quadriceps action to maintain stability. Chronic overload of the knee was the cause for knee pain (6, 8).

Electromyographic study of the left limb revealed premature onset of phasic activity in the gastrocnemius/soleus and in the medial hamstrings, and stance phase prolongation of the vastus medialis and vastus lateralis (Fig. 9.2B). Tracings of film from the front camera showed upper-lower body segment disproportion due to growth inhibition of the lower limbs and exaggerated knee flexion (Fig. 9.2C). Preoperative measurements of movements showed left knee flexion at 60° or more during stance phase (Fig. 9.2D). The preoperative problem was summarized as muscle imbalance of the knee with chronic overstretching of the quadriceps muscle and patellar tendon and contracture of the hamstring muscles. The precipitating cause was overlengthening of the heel cords. Distal tendon lengthening of all hamstring muscles was the treatment of choice at this time.

Improvement of lower extremity alignment can be seen in tracings of movie film 1 year postoperatively (Fig. 9.2, E and F). The measured improvement in knee motion throughout the gait cycle is evident in the graph of knee flexion extension (Fig. 9.2D).

Floor reaction measurements showed deficient push-off (second peak vertical force) before and after surgery (10, 11) (Fig. 9.2G). The cause of weakness in push-off was surgical overlengthening of the heel cord. The preoperative center of pressure distribution of the right leg was in an equinus pattern. The postoperative pattern of progression of center of pressure was distributed more normally. The left lower extremity demonstrated an equinus pattern of center of pressure distribution preoperatively and a calcaneal pattern in the postoperative recording. This change was attributed to improvement in knee posture which unmasked the previous overlengthening of the triceps surae. The bent knee posture with excessive dorsiflexion effectively took up the slack in the triceps surae. When the knee straightened, some muscle efficiency at the ankle was lost.

Knee flexion torque dropped sharply after surgery (Fig. 9.2H). Ankle

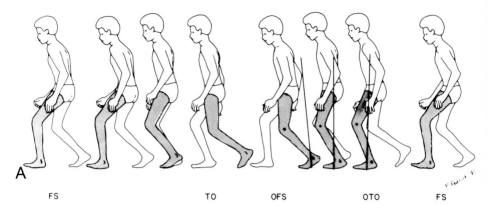

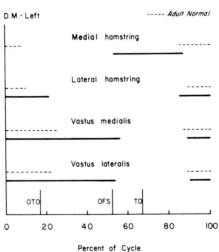

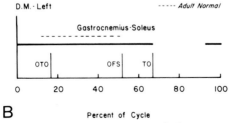

Figure 9.2. (*A* and *B*) Patient D.M.: spastic diplegia at 16 years. (*A*) Film tracings from side camera with force line superimposed during single-limb support. (See Fig. 9.1 for abbreviations.) (*B*) Phase electromyograms pre- and postoperatively with adult normal values for comparison.

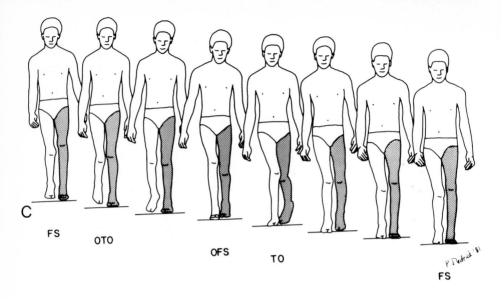

C

FS

OTO

OFS

TO

P. Dedrick '81

FS

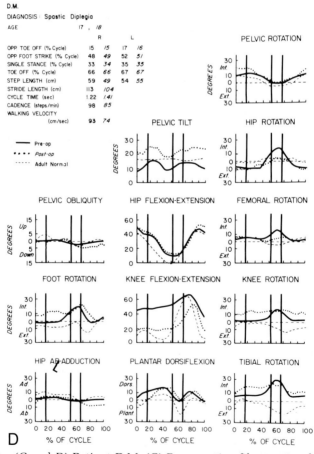

D.M.

DIAGNOSIS: Spastic Diplegia

AGE   17 , 18

	R		L	
OPP. TOE OFF (% Cycle)	15	15	17	16
OPP. FOOT STRIKE (% Cycle)	48	49	52	51
SINGLE STANCE (% Cycle)	33	34	35	35
TOE OFF (% Cycle)	66	66	67	67
STEP LENGTH (cm)	59	49	54	55
STRIDE LENGTH (cm)	113	104		
CYCLE TIME (sec)	1.22	1.41		
CADENCE (steps/min)	98	85		
WALKING VELOCITY (cm/sec)	93	74		

——— Pre-op

• • • • Post-op

- - - - Adult Normal

PELVIC ROTATION

PELVIC TILT

HIP ROTATION

PELVIC OBLIQUITY

HIP FLEXION-EXTENSION

FEMORAL ROTATION

FOOT ROTATION

KNEE FLEXION-EXTENSION

KNEE ROTATION

HIP AB-ADDUCTION

PLANTAR DORSIFLEXION

TIBIAL ROTATION

D   % OF CYCLE   % OF CYCLE   % OF CYCLE

Figure 9.2. (C and D) Patient D.M. (C) Preoperative film tracing from front camera. (D) Linear measurements and joint angles pre- and postoperatively with adult normal values for comparison.

138

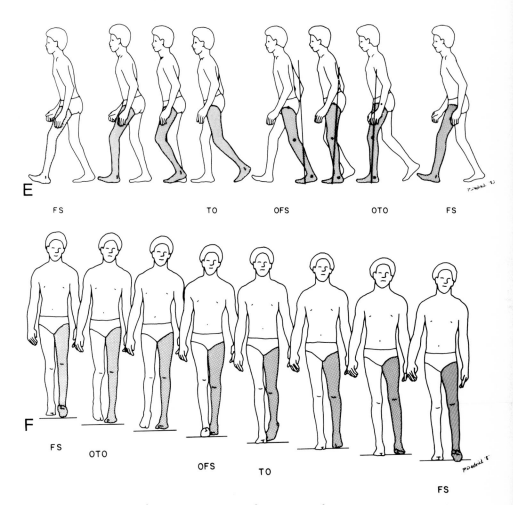

E

FS   TO   OFS   OTO   FS

F

FS   OTO   OFS   TO   FS

Figure 9.2. (*E* and *F*) Patient D.M. Film tracings from 1-year postoperative films, side camera (*E*), with superimposition of force line during single-limb support; front camera (*F*).

dorsiflexion torque also dropped because of slackness in the triceps surae secondary to reduced knee flexion. The overall effect of the surgery was marked improvement in appearance and total correction of chronic knee strain symptoms. The objectives of the corrective surgery were achieved. However, prevention of this deformity is an attainable goal and depends primarily upon avoidance of bilateral heel cord overlengthening. Also, hip and knee contractures should be treated before tendoachilles lengthening is attempted (8).

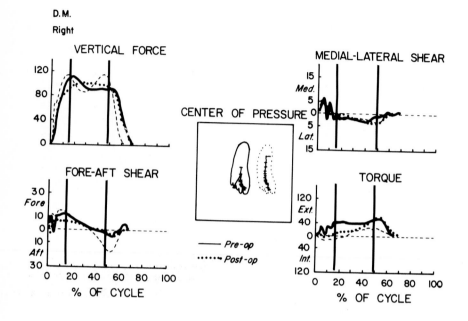

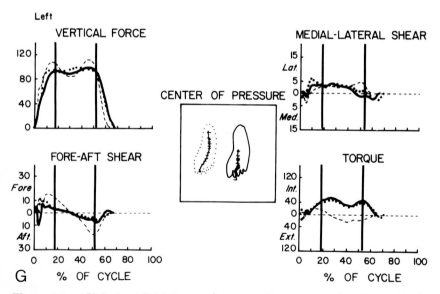

Figure 9.2. (G) Patient D.M. Force plate recordings pre- and postoperatively with adult normal values for comparison.

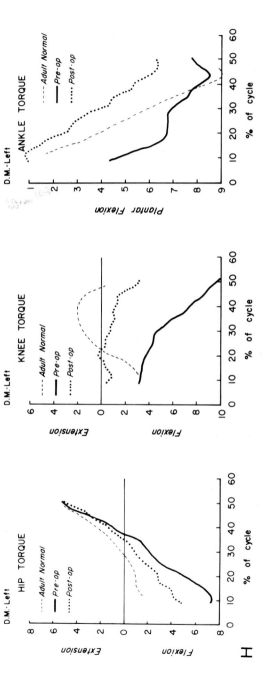

Figure 9.2. (H) Patient D.M. Normalized hip, knee and ankle torques pre- and postoperatively with adult normal values for comparison.

Spastic Quadriplegia

Patient H.U., a 9-year-old girl, was referred for gait analysis because of difficulties with walking, fatiguability and impaired range of ambulation. Adductor and proximal hamstring releases were performed at 6 years of age. The patient could walk only a short distance with bilateral short-leg braces and walker. Voluntary muscle control in the lower extremities was extremely poor, and she had problems with her hands as well. There were 5° bilateral hip flexion contractures, 10° bilateral knee flexion contractures and equinus contractures of 10°. Straight leg-raising was 60/60, and a Babinski test was positive bilaterally. Support was required for sitting balance. The patient walked in equinus and had trouble bending her knees while walking.

Film tracings from the side camera show a forward trunk lean, bilateral equinus, and limited knee flexion during swing phase (Fig. 9.3A). Film tracings from the front camera point up the effort required to clear the left foot in swing phase as evidenced by forceful extension of the left elbow (Fig. 9.3B). This patient's problems were related to both instability in stance phase and stiffness of the knees which interfered with advancement of the limbs in swing phase.

Walking velocity was 14 cm per second, cadence was 73 steps per minute, and step length was 8 cm on the right and 15 cm on the left (Fig. 9.3C). Ambulation at this speed wastes energy, consumes time, and is only useful for limited movement about the house. All movements were abnormal (Fig. 9.3C), but excessive anterior pelvic tilt, limited extension of the hip, limited knee flexion in swing phase and marked equinus throughout the entire cycle should be noted particularly. The most striking timing abnormality was severe restriction of single limb stance. The right limb was unsupported for only 9% of the walk cycle and the left for 13%. A child with this degree of motor impairment depends primarily on wheelchair mobility and extensive efforts to encourage ambulation are unwarranted. However, preservation of household ambulation is desirable.

Electromyographic study of the right medial hamstrings, rectus femoris and vastus lateralis showed phasic prolongation in stance phase (Fig. 9.3D). The rectus femoris was active through all of swing phase, interfering with normal knee flexion (9). Electromyographic recording of the gastrocnemius/soleus, tibialis posterior and tibialis anterior showed phasic prolongation in the gastrocnemius/soleus and tibialis posterior, and premature onset of phasic activity in the gastrocnemius/soleus. Prolonged muscle activity in all of the muscles is common in severely involved quadriplegic patients. This prolonged muscle activity undoubtedly explains the high energy output in such

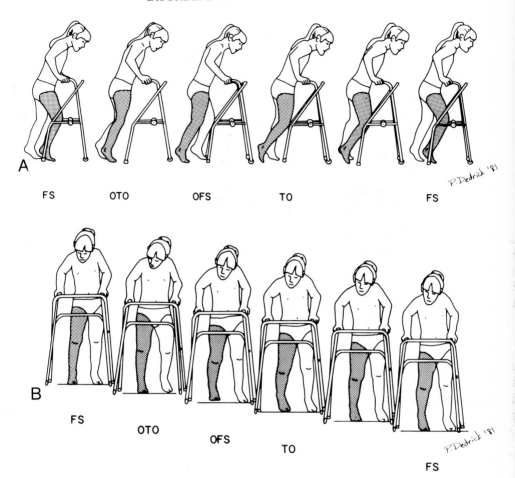

Figure 9.3. (A and B) Patient H.U., age 9 years: spastic quadriplegia. Preoperative film tracings from side (A) and front (B) camera. (See Fig. 9.1 for abbreviations.)

subjects. An energy study was not done on this patient, but reports of oxygen consumption in similar patients reveal incredibly high energy requirements for ambulation (3).

The conclusions drawn from the study were that surgical lengthening of the rectus femoris tendons was indicated to relieve knee stiffness (9), and that bilateral heel cord lengthening was required to allow more stable weight bearing. This patient has not had a postoperative gait study, but the clinic record indicates postoperative improvement in stability and ease of walking.

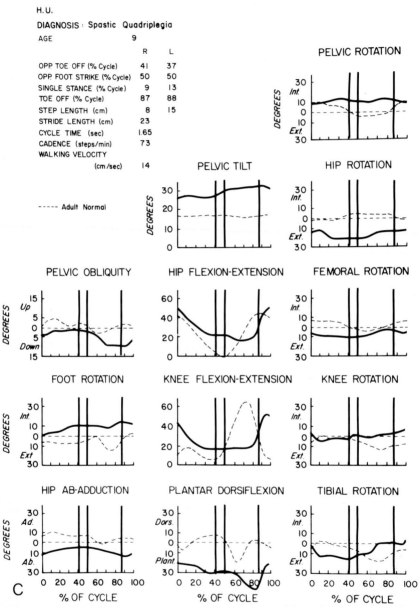

Figure 9.3. (C) Patient H.U. Linear measurements and joint angles, right lower extremity, with adult normal values for comparison.

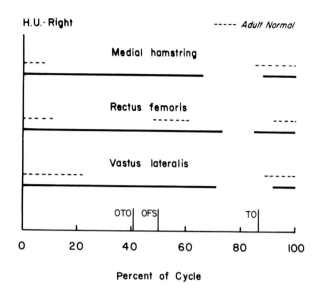

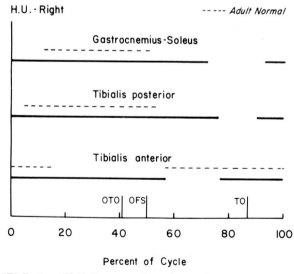

D

Figure 9.3. (*D*) Patient H.U. Preoperative phase electromyograms with adult normal values for comparison.

PROGRESSIVE DISORDER: FAMILIAL SPASTIC DIPLEGIA (4)

Patient M.D.F., an 8½-year-old girl, was a product of full-term pregnancy and breech delivery with no evidence of neurologic insult at birth. Her walking was delayed until age 5 years, but other developmental milestones were normal. The family history was significant, since three cousins on the father's side had lower limb spasticity. While the parents believed that the child showed progressive improvement, physicians who followed this child and other members of the family felt that the spasticity was slowly getting worse. The gait was characterized by adduction, internal rotation at the hips, and equinus of the ankles with no heel contact throughout the walk cycle. With the knees extended, dorsiflexion of the right ankle was −5° and −10° in the left ankle.

Film tracings from the side camera revealed flexed hip, flexed knee, and equinus ankle posture throughout the majority of the gait cycle (Fig. 9.4A). Film tracings from the front camera showed scissoring, internal rotation at the hip, equinus, bilateral gluteus medius lurch and arm posturing (Fig. 9.4B). Abnormal movements included increased hip and knee flexion, severe equinus, and marked internal rotation of the hip (Fig. 9.4C).

Floor reaction measurements (Fig. 9.4D) of the right lower extremity revealed diminished loading, diminished forward and aft shear, increased medial shear, and total concentration of center of pressure in the forefoot. Measurements of the left lower extremity revealed increased loading, diminished aft shear, oscillation of medial to lateral shear, and total concentration of center of pressure in the forward portion of the foot. Electromyography demonstrated premature onset of phasic activity in the right medial hamstrings and gastrocnemius/soleus, and phasic prolongation in stance of the medial and lateral hamstrings and tibialis anterior (Fig. 9.4E). Following gait analysis, bilateral tendoachilles lengthening and bilateral distal hamstring lengthening were performed. Examination 8 months after surgery revealed improvement in walking.

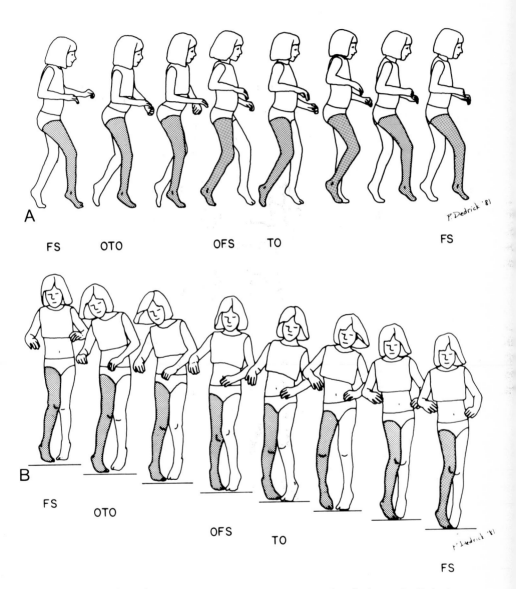

Figure 9.4. (A and B) Patient M.D.F., age 8½ years: familial spastic diplegia. Preoperative film tracings from side (A) and front (B) camera. (See Fig. 9.1 for abbreviations.)

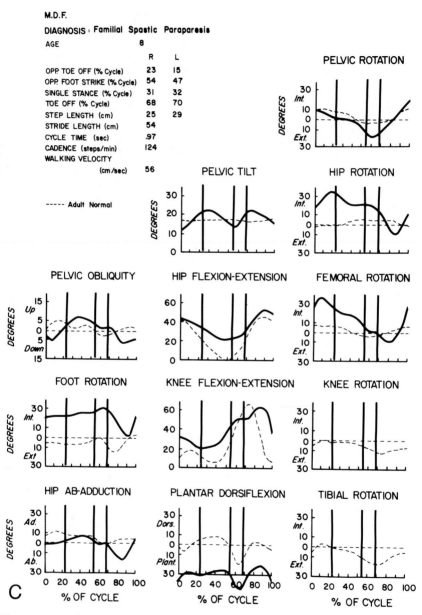

Figure 9.4. (C) Patient M.D.F. Linear measurements and joint angles, right lower extremity, preoperatively.

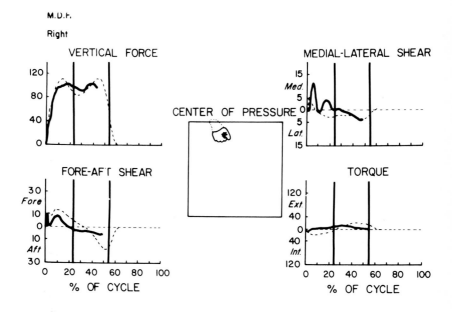

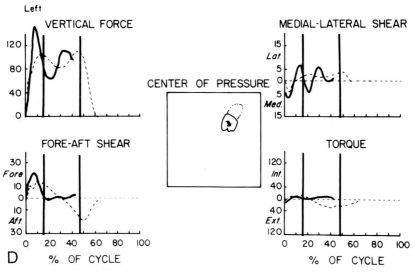

Figure 9.4.   (D) Patient M.D.F. Force plate recordings.

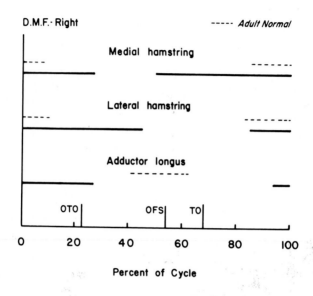

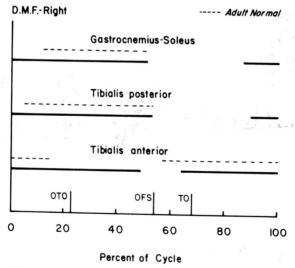

Figure 9.4.   (E) Patient M.D.F. Preoperative phase electromyograms with adult normal values for comparison.

DISCUSSION

The four examples cited in this chapter are insufficient to cover the full scope of gait analysis application to diseases of motor control. They do serve, however, as examples of common gait disorders in cerebral palsy and emphasize the benefits of objective analysis which aids in the decision process for treatment and post-treatment assessment (5, 7–9). Progress in the treatment of cerebral palsy will come from greater understanding of the pathophysiology of the disease, as well as from pooled prospective studies evaluating treatment from multiple laboratory centers. Collaboration and pooling of data will strengthen knowledge about the efficacy of various kinds of treatment.

References

1. Bax MCO: Terminology and classification of cerebral palsy. *Dev Med Child Neurol* 6:295–297, 1964.
2. Bleck EE: *Orthopedic Management of Cerebral Palsy.* Philadelphia, W.B. Saunders, 1979.
3. Campbell J, Bull J: Energetics of walking in cerebral palsy. *Orthop Clin North Am* 9:374–377, 1978.
4. Ford FR: *Diseases of the Nervous System in Infancy, Childhood and Adolescence,* ed. 6. Springfield, Ill., Charles C Thomas, 1973, pp 22–30.
5. Perry J, Hoffer MD: Preoperative and postoperative dynamic electromyography as an aid in planning tendon transfers in children with cerebral palsy. *J Bone Joint Surg* 59A:531–537, 1977.
6. Perry J, Antonelli D, Ford W: Analysis of knee-joint forces during flexed knee stance. *J Bone Joint Surg* 57A:961–967, 1975.
7. Sutherland DH: Gait analysis in cerebral palsy: review article. *Dev Med Child Neurol* 30:807–813, 1978.
8. Sutherland DH, Cooper L: The pathomechanics of progressive crouch gait in spastic diplegia. *Orthop Clin North Am* 9:143–154, 1978.
9. Sutherland DH, Larsen LJ, Mann R: Rectus femoris release in selected patients with cerebral palsy: a preliminary report. *Dev Med Child Neurol* 17:26–34, 1975.
10. Sutherland DH: Clinical use of force data. Proceedings of Gait Analysis Conference, September 1979, Long Beach, California. *Bull Prosthet Res* 18:312–316, 1981.
11. Sutherland DH, Cooper L, Daniel D: Role of the ankle plantar flexors in normal walking. *J Bone Joint Surg* 62A:354–363, 1980.

CHAPTER 10

Myopathic Disorders

INTRODUCTION

The diagnosis of myopathic disorders is based on history and physical examination, elevated serum enzyme levels, electrocardiographic and electromyographic abnormalities, and muscle biopsy. The family history is frequently positive, giving clues to the mode of inheritance. The age of onset is helpful. In general, myopathies with the earliest onset of muscle weakness are associated with the most rapid progression of weakness. For example, in Duchenne muscular dystrophy, signs of weakness may appear at 2 or 3 years of age, and the ability to walk independently ends some time between 10 and 13 years of age. The distribution of weakness may be helpful. Many of the myopathies have proximal weakness in common, such as Duchenne muscular dystrophy and limb girdle dystrophy, but two varieties produce significant distal muscle weakness—scapuloperoneal dystrophy and hereditary distal myopathy. The excellent books by Brooke and by Dubowitz describe the diagnostic features of a variety of muscle diseases (2, 4).

The problems in walking experienced by subjects with muscular dystrophy are the result of muscle weakness, not abnormal muscle control. However, myotonic dystrophy is an exception. Both muscle weakness and inability to turn off muscle contraction accompany myotonic dystrophy. In the muscle dystrophies other than the myotonic type, compensatory movements minimize the strain on weak muscle groups. In most instances, weakness is symmetrical and the gait abnormalities are symmetrical. However muscle contractures can be unequal, producing asymmetry of walking.

DUCHENNE MUSCULAR DYSTROPHY

The pathomechanics of gait in Duchenne muscular dystrophy have been scrutinized in the Motion Analysis Laboratory at Children's Hospital and Health Center in San Diego (11). Forty-six separate gait studies were analyzed in 21 ambulatory patients. Three groups—early, transitional and late—were staged on the basis of significant gait variables. Disease progression could be predicted with 91% accuracy by three variables: cadence, dorsiflexion in swing, and anterior pelvic tilt. Patients in the *early* group manifested a positive Gower's sign, but gait changes were subtle, consisting of slightly increased hip flexion in swing, decreased ankle dorsiflexion in swing, and reduction in cadence. The force line moved in front of the knee center, early in single-limb support. In the *transitional* stage, anterior pelvic tilt was exaggerated, cadence was further reduced, and foot drop in swing phase was increased. Shoulder sway was noted as compensation for gluteus medius weakness. The base of support widened and the force line remained behind the hip joint and in front of the knee joint throughout single-limb support. In the *late* stage, work output expanded, cadence continued to drop, shoulder sway increased further, and the base support widened. The force line remained close to the center of the hip and in front of the knee throughout all of the single-limb support. Soon after the beginning of the late stage, the patient found walking increasingly more difficult, fell more often and expressed anxiety about falling.

To illustrate the changes in gait characteristic of different stages of this disease, tracings of movie film were made from three selected gait studies of patient R.C. Figure 10.1A (early stage) shows film tracings from a study performed at age 5 years. The force line was behind the knee only briefly in single-limb support. Foot-strike was characterized by flat foot weight acceptance. In Figure 10.1B, (transitional stage) film tracings from the study of the same subject at 7 years and 6 months of age showed increased lordosis, posterior alignment of the upper extremities, maintenance of the force line in front of the knee during and through or behind the hip joint throughout all of single-limb support. These changes in the force line with respect to the joint centers indicated that compensatory changes in the center of mass were being used to preserve the stability at the hip and knee. Maintenance of the force line behind the hip and in front of the knee indicated that the gluteus maximus and quadriceps muscles were not sufficiently strong to resist hip flexion torque or knee flexion torque. The next sequence, Figure 10.1C (late stage), was from a study at age 8 years, 2 months. The gait was labored. The force line was maintained through the hip joint and in front of the knee joint at all times, and the step length was extremely restricted. At this stage, walking was precarious and falls were frequent.

Movement abnormalities as seen from the front are illustrated for the same subject. In the *early* stage (age 5 years), Figure 10.2A shows only slight increase in arm abduction and slight widening of the base of support. In the *transitional* stage (Fig. 10.2B —7 years, 11 months) shoulder sway and arm abduction in stance phase were increased due to greater weakness of the gluteus medius. The width of base was expanded and there was some beginning exaggeration of internal rotation at the hip. In the *late* stage (age 8 years, 2 months), Figure 10.2C, walking was awkward; the arms were held in wide abduction

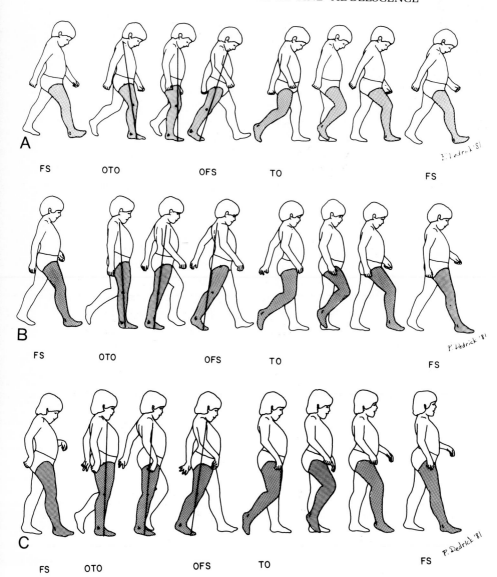

Figure 10.1. (A–C) Patient R.C.: Duchenne muscular dystrophy. Film tracings from right side camera: (A) early impairment (5 years), (B) transitional stage (7 years, 6 months), and (C) late stage (8 years, 2 months). Force lines are superimposed on right lower extremity during period of single limb support. Notice that force line becomes more vertical with increasing impairment, and hip and knee joint centers are brought closer to force line. (FS = foot-strike, OTO = opposite toe-off, OFS = opposite foot-strike, TO = toe-off.)

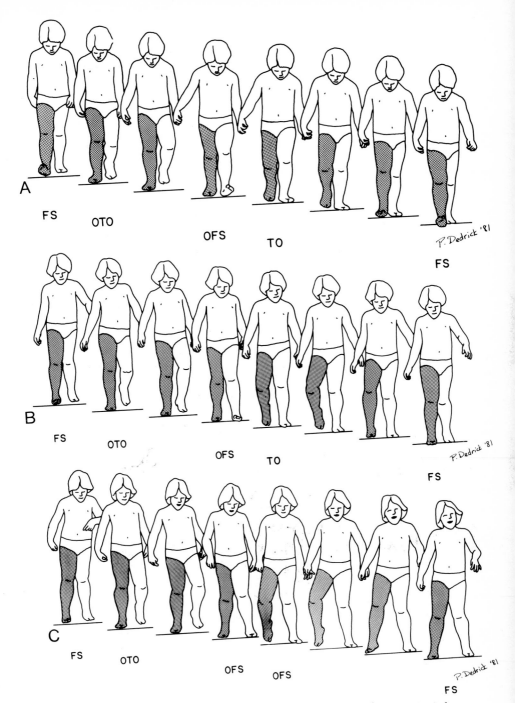

Figure 10.2. (A–C) Patient R.C. Tracings (frontal view) of one gait cycle at (A) early stage (5 years), (B) transitional stage (7 years, 11 months), and (C) late stage (8 years, 2 months). Increasing shoulder sway, ankle spread, arm abduction, and internal rotation with increasing stages of impairment can be seen. (See Fig. 10.1 for abbreviations.)

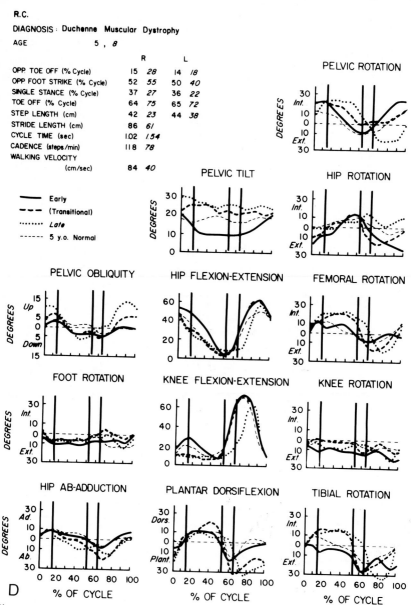

Figure 10.2. (D) Patient R.C. Joint angle rotations during early, transitional and late stages are compared with normal values for age 5 years. Linear measurements for subject R.C. are for early and transitional stages.

in stance phase; and the feet were wide apart in double support. Shoulder sway was pronounced due to weakness of the gluteus medius. Internal rotation of the hip in stance phase was present. This is often a hallmark of the late stage of walking impairment.

The changes in joint motion can be appreciated by inspection of the joint angle curves for the same subject during early, transitional and late stages of walking impairment (Fig. 10.2D). The average joint angle rotations for 5-year-old normal subjects provide a comparison. There was less than the usual degree of anterior pelvic tilt during the early stage, but this was followed by progressive increase in anterior pelvic tilt in the transitional and late stages. In the transitional and late stages, the knee flexion/extension joint angle showed exaggerated knee flexion in swing phase and progressive loss of knee extension in stance phase. In both transitional and late stages, the knee remained in an extended posture throughout the stance phase. Flat foot-strike occurred at all stages of walking impairment, but increasing loss of ankle dorsiflexion in swing phase was observed with the progression of walking impairment. Increase in pelvic obliquity was another abnormality which characterized progression of walking impairment.

Following the last study at age 8 years, 2 months, this patient was placed in polypropylene knee-ankle-foot orthoses with anterior tension band quadriceps assist. These orthoses offered greater knee stability, thereby protecting against falls. When weight increased and weakness progressed, knee locks for the braces became mandatory. Nonetheless, contractures were avoided and ambulation was preserved until age 12 years.

In Duchenne dystrophy, final dependence upon a wheelchair for mobility usually begins by about the age of 10 years. The duration of independent ambulation can be extended for an additional 2–5 years by well-coordinated efforts, including physical therapy, long-leg bracing, contracture release when walking becomes labored, immediate reambulation in long-leg casts and then long-leg brace (1, 3, 5–10). Research findings in this laboratory lend support to the hypothesis that contractures can be minimized or prevented by earlier bracing for quadriceps insufficiency. If braces are withheld until walking is labored, it is usually necessary to release contractures before appropriate bracing can be applied.

LIMB GIRDLE DYSTROPHY

Patient A.A., a 19-year-old youth with limb girdle dystrophy, had marked weakness and atrophy of the upper arms, hips and thighs. His

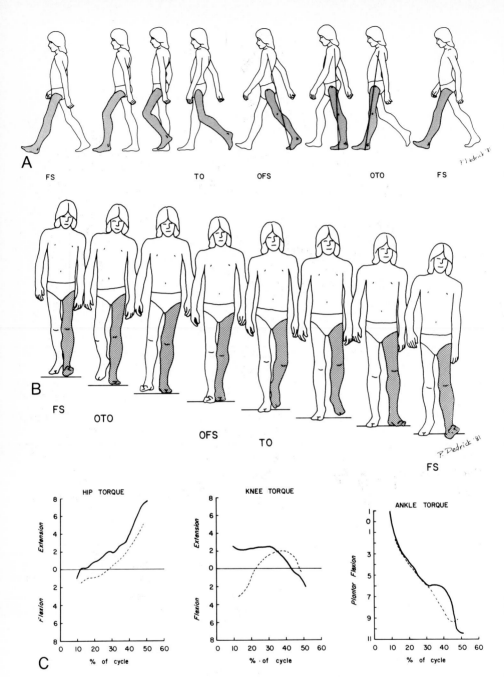

A

FS   TO   OFS   OTO   FS

B

FS
    OTO
            OFS
                    TO

                                                              FS

HIP TORQUE   KNEE TORQUE   ANKLE TORQUE

C

Figure 10.3. (A–C) Patient A.A.: limb girdle dystrophy. (A) Film tracings from left side camera with force line superimposed during single limb support. (B) Film tracings, frontal view. Cycle proceeds from left to right. (C) Hip, knee and ankle torque compared with mean of normal subjects. Torque values are normalized by adjustment for body weight and height. Thus torque units are eliminated. Solid lines—patient A.A. Broken lines—adult normal values. (See Fig. 10.1 for abbreviations.)

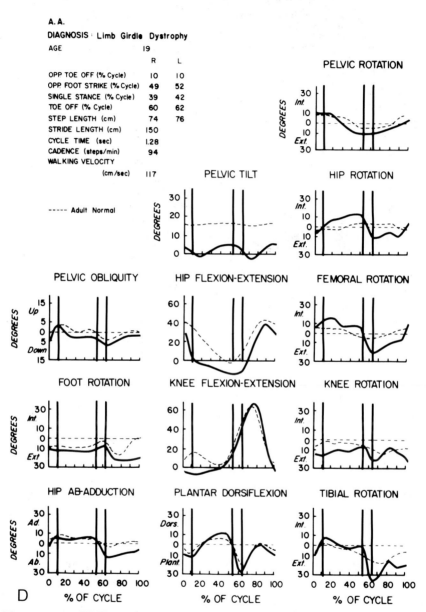

Figure 10.3. (D) Patient A.A.: Linear measurements and joint angle rotations at 19 years of age.

abdominal muscles were strong enough to permit him to do multiple sit-ups, but stair climbing and running were difficult. Minimal hip abduction contractures were present. Muscle testing demonstrated gluteus maximum strength of 2+/3 and quadriceps strength of 4−/ 4−. Film tracings from the side camera showed increased lordosis and posterior alignment of the trunk (Fig. 10.3A). The knee was held in full extension throughout single-limb stance. The increase in lumbar lordosis and the posterior alignment of the trunk maintained the force line behind the hip joint, preventing extrinsic flexion torque (which the weak hip extensors could not resist). The force line was maintained in front of the knee, except in the last portion of single-limb stance, preventing knee extrinsic flexion torque (which the quadriceps could not resist).

The front camera view showed mild increase in shoulder sway (Fig. 10.3B). Hip, knee and ankle torque measurements on this subject compared with normal subjects are shown in Figure 10.3C. In the normal pattern, hip torque begins in flexion and passes to extension at 30% of the gait cycle. In this subject, there was a short period of flexion torque, followed by hip extension torque throughout the remainder of the walk cycle. The normal pattern of knee torque begins as flexion, passes to extension at approximately 22% of the cycle, and there is a final slight return to flexion near 50% of the cycle. In this subject, the extension torque (force line in front of the knee) persisted through the majority of single-limb stance, only changing to flexion torque at the end of the period. This exemplified a postural adaptation to relieve stress on a weak muscle group (quadriceps).

Principal movement abnormalities evident in joint angle measurements (Fig. 10.3D) were: rapid hip extension following foot strike, hyperextension of the hip in stance phase, full knee extension through-out all of the early portion of the single-limb stance, and flat foot strike. Comparison is made with average adult values.

This patient's impairment did not require bracing for quadriceps insufficiency. His weakness had progressed, but the rate of progression was slow. No treatment measures were contemplated at that time, but long-leg braces may be needed in the future.

FASCIOSCAPULOHUMERAL DYSTROPHY

K.T., an 18-year-old patient with fascioscapulohumeral dystrophy, complained that her left knee gave way and that she had some difficulty in clearing the left foot. On examination there were no significant contractures, but she could not do sit-ups. Muscle strength

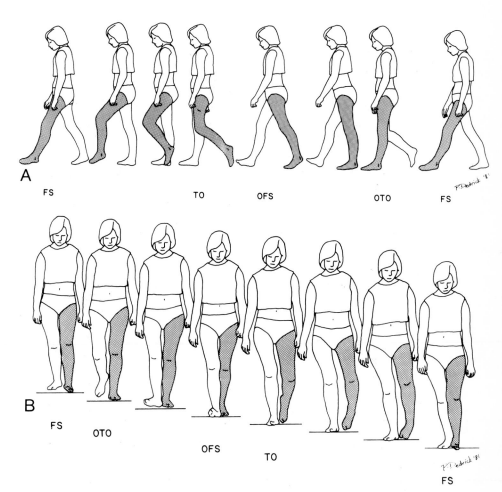

A

FS   TO   OFS   OTO   FS

B

FS   OTO   OFS   TO

FS

Figure 10.4. (*A* and *B*) Patient K.T.: fascioscapulohumeral dystrophy. (*A*) Film tracings from left side camera of one gait cycle. (*B*) Film tracings from front camera. This cycle proceeds from left to right. (See Fig. 10.1 for abbreviations.)

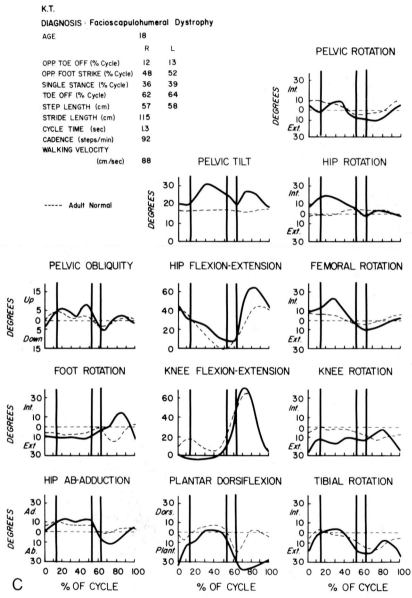

Figure 10.4.   (C) Patient K.T. Linear measurements and joint angle rotations.

was as follows:

	R/L
Hip extensors	2/3
Hip abductors	3−/3
Quadriceps	4−/3
Medial hamstrings	4/4
Lateral hamstrings	4/4
Tibialis anterior	4/2+
Extensor hallucis longus	3/2
Extensor digitorum longus	4/3
Gastrocnemius	5/5
Tibialis posterior	4/4
Peroneus	5/4

Film tracings from the left camera (Fig. 10.4A) showed flat foot-strike, drop foot in swing phase, and exaggerated hip and knee flexion in swing phase to clear the drop foot. Front film tracings (Fig. 10.4B) demonstrated supination of the foot at foot-strike, and supination and inversion of the foot throughout early swing phase.

The joint angle values throughout the walk cycle and the linear measurements are given in Figure 10.4C. The ankle plantar flexion dorsiflexion curve showed plantar flexion at foot strike and marked drop foot in swing phase. The knee flexion/extension curve showed full knee extension throughout stance phase. The hip flexion/extension curve showed exaggerated hip flexion in swing phase to provide foot clearance. Foot rotation was normal in stance phase, but there was marked internal rotation of the foot during swing phase.

Most of this patient's complaints related to drop foot, and a polypropylene ankle-foot orthosis relieved this problem.

MYOTONIC DYSTROPHY

The diagnosis of myotonic dystrophy in patient T.H. was established in the first few weeks of life. The family history was positive for myotonic dystrophy both in the patient's mother and maternal uncle. Two siblings appeared to be free of the disease. There was some delay in the patient's developmental milestone. She could turn over at 8 months of age and sat at 14 months of age. At 16 months of age, bilateral heel cord lengthenings were performed because of equinus contractures. Braces were worn for a time following the heel cord lengthenings, but the braces were discarded and the equinus contractures recurred. At 7 years of age, there was marked weakness of the facial musculature, and the mouth was open, creating the characteristic dull facies. Diffuse muscle weakness, mild myotonia of grip in both hands and a positive Gower sign were present. There were

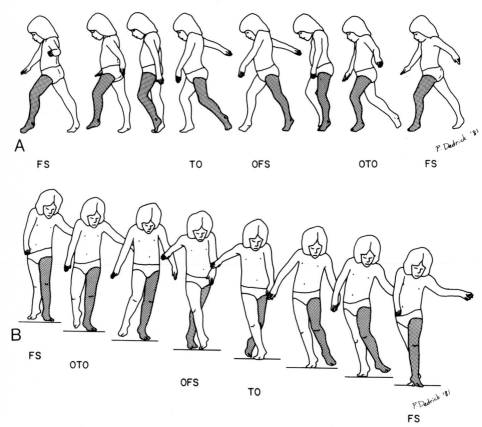

Figure 10.5. (A and B) Patient T.H.: Myotonic dystrophy. (A) Film tracings from left side camera. (B) Film tracings from front camera. Cycle proceeds from left to right. (See Fig. 10.1 for abbreviations.)

bilateral hip flexion contractures of 20°, bilateral knee flexion contractures of 20°, a 20° right equinus contracture and a left equinus contracture limiting dorsiflexion to neutral. The patient walked with a peculiar vaulting gait. Her walking cadence was 164 steps per minute—abnormally high for her age. Walking velocity was 121 cm per second, normal for her age. Stride length was 88 cm, compared with an average of 96.5 cm for her age. Tracings taken from the side camera view (Fig. 10.5A) demonstrated excessive arm swing, bilateral equinus and anterior trunk lean. Front camera views (Fig. 10.5B) showed excessive trunk sway, scissoring, and abnormal arm swing. The child gave every appearance of an impending fall, as she hurried along, staggering from step to step. The extreme abnormalities of movement were apparent in the joint angle measurements (Fig. 10.5C). Anterior pelvic tilt was exaggerated; hip extension in stance was

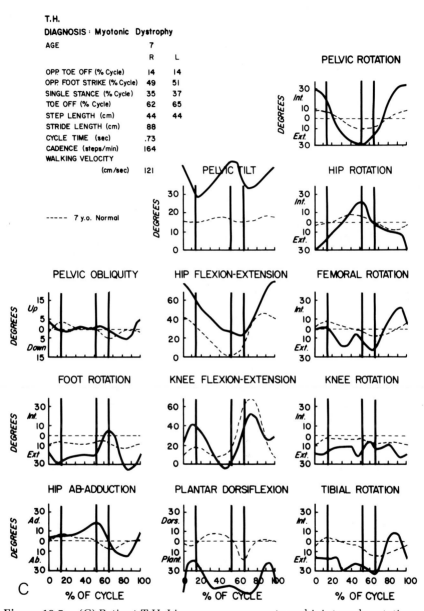

T.H.

DIAGNOSIS : Myotonic Dystrophy

AGE   7

	R	L
OPP. TOE OFF (% Cycle)	14	14
OPP. FOOT STRIKE (% Cycle)	49	51
SINGLE STANCE (% Cycle)	35	37
TOE OFF (% Cycle)	62	65
STEP LENGTH (cm)	44	44
STRIDE LENGTH (cm)	88	
CYCLE TIME (sec)	.73	
CADENCE (steps/min)	164	
WALKING VELOCITY (cm/sec)	121	

----- 7 y.o. Normal

PELVIC ROTATION

PELVIC TILT

HIP ROTATION

PELVIC OBLIQUITY

HIP FLEXION-EXTENSION

FEMORAL ROTATION

FOOT ROTATION

KNEE FLEXION-EXTENSION

KNEE ROTATION

HIP AB-ADDUCTION

PLANTAR DORSIFLEXION

TIBIAL ROTATION

C

Figure 10.5. (C) Patient T.H. Linear measurements and joint angle rotations.

diminished; severe equinus was present throughout the gait cycle; pelvic rotation was exaggerated; and there was excessive hip adduction in stance phase.

Because of technical difficulties, force data were not obtained on this patient. Serial casting with short-leg casts was done to overcome the equinus contractures. When both ankles could be brought to neutral position, polypropylene ankle-foot orthoses with anterior straps to keep the heels properly seated were provided. Walking was much improved. The patient moved to another state, and it was not possible to obtain a post-treatment gait analysis. Long-term prognosis for ambulation is guarded because of the severity of the gait abnormality and the current level of difficulty in walking.

References

1. Bowker JH, Halpin PJ: Factors determining success in re-ambulation of the child with progressive muscular dystrophy. *Orthop Clin North Am* 9:431–436, 1978.
2. Brooke MH: *A Clinician's View of Neuromuscular Diseases*. Baltimore, Williams and Wilkins, 1977.
3. Curtis BH: Orthopedic management of muscular dystrophy and related disorders. *Am Acad Orthop Surgeons Instruct Course Lect* 19:78–89, 1970.
4. Dubowitz V: *Muscle Disorders in Childhood: Vol. XVI. Major Problems in Clinical Pediatrics*. Philadelphia, W. B. Saunders, 1978.
5. Johnson EW: The care and management of the child with muscular dystrophy. *Dev Med Child Neurol* 16:396–397, 1974.
6. Johnson EW, Eyring EJ, Burnett C: Surgery in muscular dystrophy. *JAMA* 222:1056–1057, 1972.
7. Miller J: Management of muscular dystrophy. *J Bone Joint Surg* 49A:1205–1211, 1967.
8. Siegel IM, Miller JE, Ray RD: Subcutaneous lower limb tenotomy in treatment of pseudohypertrophic muscular dystrophy. *J Bone Joint Surg* 50A:1437–1443, 1968.
9. Spencer GE: Orthopedic care of progressive muscular dystrophy. *J Bone Joint Surg* 49A:1201–1204, 1967.
10. Spencer GE, Vignos PJ: Bracing for ambulation in childhood progressive muscular dystrophy. *J Bone Joint Surg* 44A:234–252, 1962.
11. Sutherland DH, Olshen R, Cooper LB, et al: The pathomechanics of gait in Duchenne muscular dystrophy. *Dev Med Child Neurol* 23:3–22, 1981.

CHAPTER **11**

Progressive Spinal Cord and Peripheral Nerve Disorders

INTRODUCTION

No physical examination is complete without inspection of standing and walking posture. With many diagnostic possibilities, few examiners, no matter how thorough, will think of every test for motor skeletal function. Observation of gait can call attention to obvious abnormalities which can then be systematically examined. For instance, ataxia causes instability during single-limb stance, and patients with this problem show an alternating width of the base during double-limb support. At times the swinging limb crosses the midline, while at other times ankle spread increases. The experienced observer can detect the variations in width of the base and then perform tests of tandem walking, finger-to-nose and heel-to-shin movements which are poorly handled by patients with ataxia.

A patient with Charcot-Marie-Tooth disease may exhibit lateral atrophy of the legs, cavus deformities of the feet, clawing of the toes, and swing phase equinus of the feet in walking (1). These visual observations will alert the informed examiner to obtain a history which may include complaints of slowly progressive weakness of the hands and feet and the existence of similar problems in other family members. Then the strength of the peroneal muscles and the strength of the intrinsic muscles of the hands can be examined. Tendon reflexes are usually absent. Diagnostic tests frequently show delayed motor nerve conduction velocities, and a presumptive diagnosis can be made of Charcot-Marie-Tooth disease (1, 4). As a word of caution, many neurologic disorders have some presenting features in common. The examiner must seek out family history, perform a careful neurological examination, and obtain proper laboratory tests in order to determine an accurate diagnosis. When this has been established, prognosis and genetic counseling can be given.

Thus far in this introduction, visual gait observation has been stressed. Formal gait analysis is also beneficial for the study of progressive neurologic disorders, because sequential studies provide quantitative measurements of changes over periods of time. For example, gait abnormalities in Becker's muscular dystrophy resemble Duchenne dystrophy, but gait deterioration in Becker's dystrophy progresses slowly. The two types can be distinguished by systemati-

167

cally measuring gait parameters over an appropriate time span. Such studies are ongoing in this laboratory for the disease categories included in this chapter, but enough studies have not yet been accumulated to make a definitive statement on progression patterns.

SPINAL MUSCULAR ATROPHY

Patient C.H. began to toe-walk at 11 years of age. A pediatric neurologist examined him at 14 years of age and noted proximal weakness and heel cord contractures. Creatinine phosphokinase was 6700 IU/ml, and muscle biopsy was interpreted to show both neuropathic and myopathic elements. A trial course of prednisone made no significant improvement in the patient's strength, and a diagnosis of Kugelberg-Welander's disease was made (2, 5, 6).

By the time the patient was 16½ years of age, he could climb only six steps before fatiguing. His heels did not contact the floor during standing or walking, and he could not run. The abdominal muscles were weak, and there was proximal weakness of the upper extremities.

Lower extremity muscle strength:

	Right	Left
Hip flexion	4	4
Gluteus maximus	2+	3
Quadriceps	2+	3
Tibialis anterior	2+	3
Extensor hallucis longus	4	4
Extensor digitorum longus	3	4
Gastrocnemius/soleus	5	5
Tibialis posterior	5	5
Peroneals	5	4

Fixed equinus contractures of 30° were present.

The treatment dilemma posed was that correction of the equinus contractures by lengthening would weaken the gastrocnemius and soleus, and there was danger of converting the patient from a toe walker who could walk independently to a flat foot walker who requires full-length braces. However, the contractures required treatment, since they interfered with function. The plan chosen was to apply short-leg casts, changing them every 2 weeks to gradually lengthen the triceps surae. The casting was effective, reducing the equinus contractures to 15°. Bilateral tendoachilles lengthening then brought the ankles to neutral position. Gait studies were done prior to heel cord lengthening. At the time of a postoperative gait study, the right ankle could be brought to neutral, but the left ankle showed an equinus contracture of 10°. This equinus recurrence was attributed to the patient's failure to wear braces regularly. He was a young man of engaging personality and above average intelligence, but apparently the fear of contracture recurrence was not sufficient to motivate consistent use of the braces. He felt much improved by surgery, and postoperative gait study confirmed this impression.

Film tracings from the right side camera (Fig. 11.1A) showed absent heel contact for both feet throughout the walk cycle and short step length. Film tracings from the front camera revealed a slight increase in lateral sway (gluteus medius lurch—Fig. 11.1C). Cadence and walking velocity were slow, and step length was restricted to 54 cm on the right and 58 cm on the left (Fig. 11.1E). Since movements of the two lower extremities were similar, measurements of the right only are shown. There was lack of full extension of the hip in stance phase. The knee remained fully extended in stance, and the ankle remained in equinus of more than 25° throughout the gait cycle. Hip internal

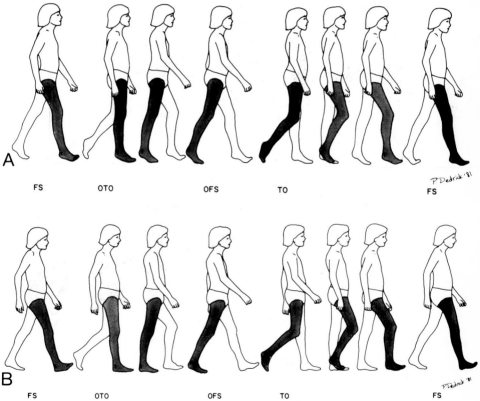

Figure 11.1. (A and B) Patient C.H., age 16½ years: Kugelberg-Welander variety of spinal muscular atrophy. (A) Preoperative tracings from right camera film. (B) Postoperative 1 year after serial casting and bilateral tendoachilles lengthening. (FS = foot-strike, OTO = opposite toe-off, OFS = opposite foot-strike, and TO = toe-off.)

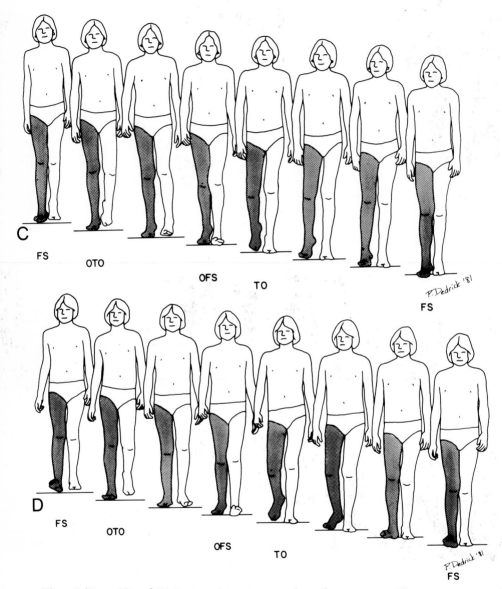

Figure 11.1. (*C* and *D*) Patient C.H. Tracings from front camera film, preoperative (*C*) and postoperative (*D*).

rotation and adduction in stance were exaggerated. Increased initial loading, increased forward shear, and an equinus pattern of center of pressure progression were noted in the right lower limb, with slightly diminished initial loading, increased internal torque, and an equinus pattern of center of pressure for the left lower extremity (Fig. 11.1F).

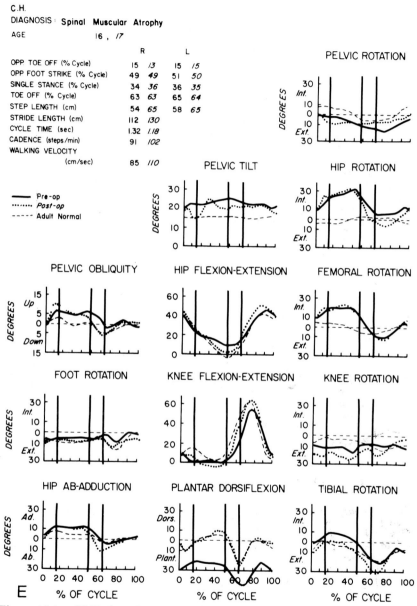

C.H.
DIAGNOSIS: Spinal Muscular Atrophy
AGE   16 , /7

	R		L	
OPP. TOE OFF (% Cycle)	15	/3	15	/5
OPP. FOOT STRIKE (% Cycle)	49	49	51	50
SINGLE STANCE (% Cycle)	34	36	36	35
TOE OFF (% Cycle)	63	63	65	64
STEP LENGTH (cm)	54	65	58	65
STRIDE LENGTH (cm)	112	/30		
CYCLE TIME (sec)	1.32	/.18		
CADENCE (steps/min)	91	/02		
WALKING VELOCITY (cm/sec)	85	//0		

—— Pre-op
········ Post-op
- - - - Adult Normal

PELVIC ROTATION

PELVIC TILT

HIP ROTATION

PELVIC OBLIQUITY

HIP FLEXION-EXTENSION

FEMORAL ROTATION

FOOT ROTATION

KNEE FLEXION-EXTENSION

KNEE ROTATION

HIP AB-ADDUCTION

PLANTAR DORSIFLEXION

TIBIAL ROTATION

E   % OF CYCLE   % OF CYCLE   % OF CYCLE

Figure 11.1.   (E) Patient C.H. Pre- and postoperative linear measurements and joint angle rotations of the right lower extremity.

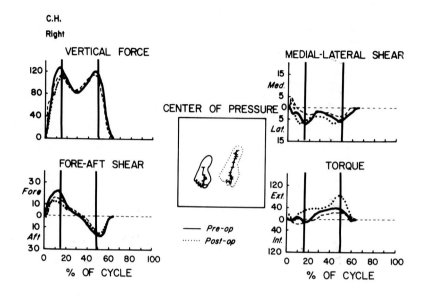

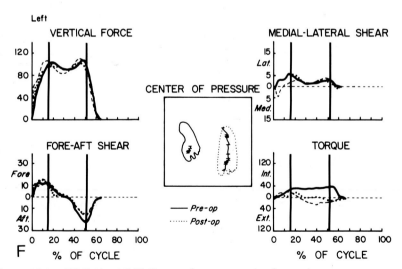

Figure 11.1. (*F*) Patient C.H. Pre- and postoperative force plate measurements with normal adult values (*dotted line*) for comparison.

Marked improvements followed casting and heel-cord lengthening. Film tracings from the side camera showed normal heel-strike and improved step length (Fig. 11.1B). Film tracings from the front camera confirmed restoration of heel-strike. The mild gluteus medius sway did not change (Fig. 11.1D). Cadence and velocity increased after surgery, as did step length. Right step length measured 65 cm (20% increase), while left step length measured 65 cm (12% increase). Hip rotation remained the same, but hip extension in stance phase became normal, and ankle motion returned to a normal pattern (Fig. 11.1E).

In the torce measurements (Fig. 11.1F), initial vertical force and forward shear which increased preoperatively were normal after surgery. Center of pressure distribution changed from an equinus pattern to a relatively normal heel-toe pattern.

For the left lower extremity, the primary changes were in center of pressure; relatively normal center of pressure progression was recorded in the postoperative study (Fig. 11.1F).

A second patient, J.D., with a slightly different expression of Kugelberg-Welander's disease, was brought to his family doctor at the age of 2, because of waddling gait. The family was told that no abnormalities were present. Between 2 and 3, the child demonstrated inability to climb stairs, step over objects, run, hop, or jump. He walked with a waddling gait and needed to push his hands on his knees when getting up from the floor. He was a toe-walker as well. Examination revealed 10° left hip flexion contracture, and knee flexion contractures, 10/10. There was weakness in the musculature below the knee; tibialis anterior was 3/3; extensor hallucis longus, 3/3; gastrocnemius/soleus, 4/4; tibialis posterior, 4/4. Clonus was absent, but right and left Babinski tests were positive. Fasciculations were numerous in the muscles of the shoulders and back, and there was wasting of the intrinsic muscles of the left hand. Deep tendon reflexes were absent. Mild scoliosis was noted. The diagnosis of Kugelberg-Welander's disease was based on the progressive course and evidence of lower motor neuron involvement.

A gait study was performed when the patient was 8 years old to serve as a baseline for future comparisons. Foot contact was made with the forefoot, and the position of equinus was maintained throughout the cycle. Hyperlordosis was evident (Fig. 11.2A). Film tracings from the front camera showed a variable base of support, as shown by differing ankle spread at FS, OFS, and FS (Fig. 11.2B). Abduction movements of the arms suggested either gluteus medius lurch or balancing movements.

The cadence was normal for age, but walking velocity was low at 83 cm per second (Fig. 11.2C). Step lengths were symmetrical. Abnor-

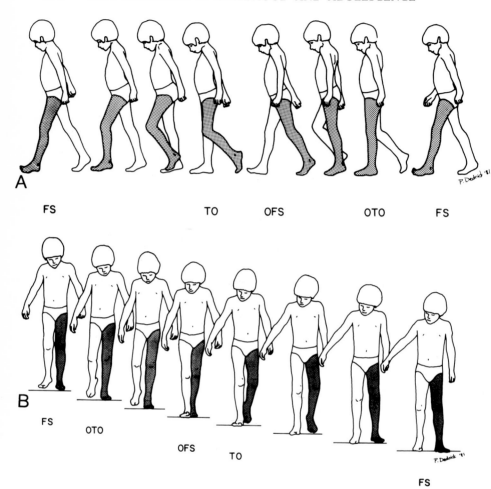

Figure 11.2. (*A* and *B*) Patient J.D., age 8 years: Kugelberg-Welander variety of spinal muscular atrophy. Tracings from left side (*A*) and front (*B*) camera film. (See Fig. 11.1 for abbreviations.)

mal movements included increased anterior pelvic tilt, diminished hip extension in stance phase, equinus throughout most of the gait cycle, and increased internal rotation of the femur.

Force plate studies (not shown) demonstrated increased forward shear and an equinus pattern of center of pressure with total concentration in the front of the foot. Both limbs demonstrated a similar pattern.

This child was subsequently placed in bilateral ankle-foot orthoses to prevent development of fixed contractures. A repeat gait study was done at 12½ years of age. This showed a drop in cadence, velocity and stride length, and an equinovarus alignment of the right foot. The

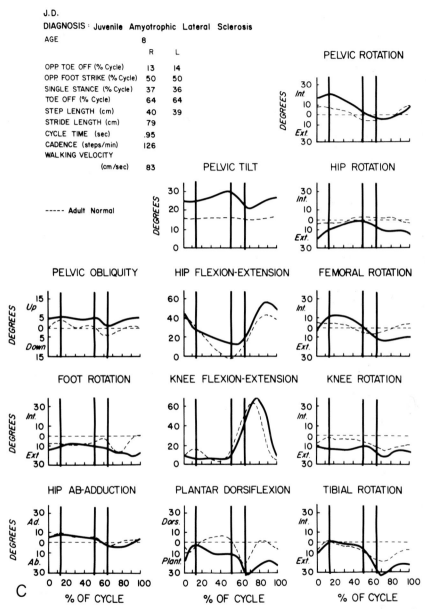

Figure 11.2.   (C) Patient J.D. Linear measurements and joint angle rotations, right lower extremity; adult normal values are given for comparison (*dotted line*).

patient exhibited signs of balance problems and developed a scoliosis which required bracing. Consideration was given to long-leg bracing to provide greater stability. Following this study, care was transferred to another institution. A current report from the neurologist indicates that the scoliosis has not increased. The patient is able to walk about the house, but is not strong enough to walk any distance.

In the two cases presented, the first patient's clinical course was characteristic of juvenile muscular atrophy (Kugelberg-Welander's disease) (6). The second patient was diagnosed as having juvenile amyotrophic lateral sclerosis, until his clinical course prompted reassessment. Because of the variability of expression of Kugelberg-Welander's disease, a firm prognosis is not possible. However, many patients are using a wheelchair in the third decade. An ongoing treatment program minimizes functional impairment, and multiple services available in a well-developed muscle disease clinic are advantageous for patients with this disorder.

CHARCOT-MARIE-TOOTH DISEASE

Patient G.M., an 11½-year-old girl, complained of painful feet and increasing discomfort on wearing shoes. Her mother observed that her walking had changed, and she could not run well. The patient's sister, father, and paternal uncle experienced similar problems.

Cavovarus deformities of both feet, mild equinus contractures, and clawing of the toes were present. It was impossible for the patient to walk on her heels. When asked to rise from the floor, she used the right hand on the right knee for support. Muscular atrophy was most obvious in the region of the lateral muscle compartment of the legs.

Muscle strength:

	Right	Left
Tibialis anterior	3+	3+
Peroneals	4	4

Results of an electromyographic study which included conduction velocities were consistent with a diagnosis of Charcot-Marie-Tooth disease. The prognosis for progression varies with the specific subtype of hereditary polyneuropathy and with the inheritance pattern (1, 4). The inheritance pattern in this case seemed to be dominant, implying a better prognosis than if it were recessive. Operative measures usually have little to offer when disease progression is rapid. In this instance, however, progression had been relatively slow; the pattern of inheritance indicated a favorable progression rate; and rehabilitative surgery presented the best possibility for improvement of function (7). A gait study was performed to give a baseline for comparison of treatment results.

Film tracings from the right side camera showed drop foot in swing phase (Fig. 11.3A). Compensatory overaction of the toe extensors can also be seen. Film tracings from the foot camera demonstrated relative inversion of the foot in swing phase and hyperextension of the toes (Fig. 11.3B). Cadence was normal, with only slightly diminished walking velocity (Fig. 11.3C). Movement abnormalities in the right foot were minor. Initial heel-strike was lost, and foot-strike occurred with the entire sole of the foot contacting the floor. Dorsiflexion in stance after this point was normal, but marked equinus appeared in swing because of tibialis anterior weakness. There was diminished hip adduction in stance phase.

Force measurements were relatively normal except for center of

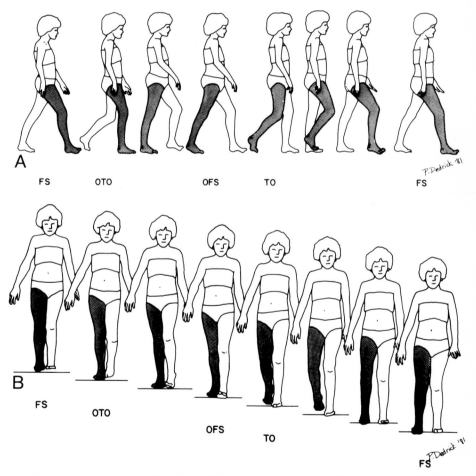

Figure 11.3. (A and B) Patient G.M., age 11½ years: Charcot-Marie-Tooth disease. Tracings of right (A) and front (B) camera film. (See Fig. 11.1 for abbreviations.)

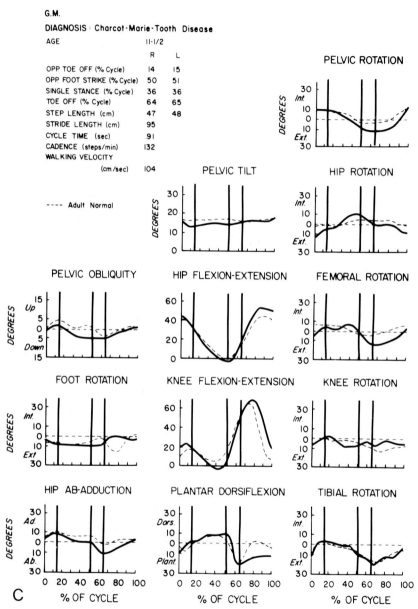

Figure 11.3.   (C) Patient G.M. Linear measurements and joint angle rotations with adult normal values (*dotted line*) for comparison.

pressure which remained concentrated in the front of the foot throughout stance (Fig. 11.3*D*).

Movement measurements in the left lower extremity (not shown) were similar, but normal ankle dorsiflexion occurred in swing phase.

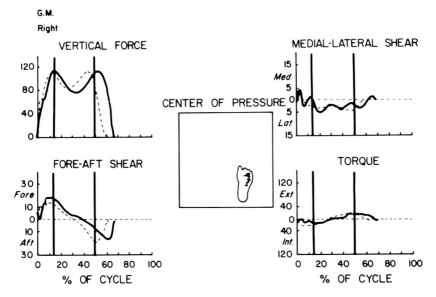

Figure 11.3. (*D*) Patient G.M. Right lower extremity force measurements. Adult normal values (*dotted line*) shown for comparison.

The first surgical procedure consisted of left plantar fasciotomy, triple arthrodesis, tendoachilles lengthening, and posterior tibial transfer through the interosseous space to the dorsum of the foot. The patient subsequently underwent right triple arthrodesis, posterior tibial transfer through the interosseous space, plantar fasciotomy, and tendoachilles lengthening.

Weight bearing was much improved by the surgeries, and the left drop foot in swing phase was corrected. Clawing of the toes persisted, and the patient is scheduled for bilateral Jones procedures to the great toe, proximal first metatarsal osteotomy, and transfers of the extensor tendons into the metatarsal necks. A comparative gait study will be performed after recovery from the final rehabilitative operations.

FRIEDREICH'S ATAXIA

Scoliosis was detected in patient P.S. at age 12 through a school screening program. Physical findings included flexible right thoracic and left lumbar scoliosis in the erect position, but disappearance of the curves in the supine posture. Positive physical findings included upper/lower body segment disproportion, with the upper segment measuring 30 inches and the lower, 35 inches. Ocular and cardiac abnormalities frequently associated with Marfan's syndrome were absent, and a urine test for homocystinuria was negative. A presumptive diagnosis of Marfan's disease (8) (forme fruste) was made, and a

Milwaukee brace was prescribed and worn to prevent progression of the scoliosis.

When the patient was 14, an orthopaedic surgeon observed mild ataxia, and neurological and pediatric neurology consultations were obtained. Mild pes cavus, ataxia, and scoliosis were the principal physical findings which suggested Friedreich's ataxia. A gait study was done primarily to serve as a baseline in case of progressive neurologic changes. When the patient reached 17 years and 9 months of age, ocular dysmetria and finger-to-nose dysmetria were noted, as well as marked ataxia in walking. Romberg's sign was positive, and deep tendon reflexes were absent. One year later, the patient exhibited dysarthria, severe ataxia with lurching, staggering gait, and bilateral foot drop, with weakness and intrinsic muscle atrophy of the hands and feet. Vibratory sense and position sense were defective in the toes, and vibratory sense was mildly diminished in the fingers.

Findings in an electromyographic study were indeterminate. Four years later, sensory nerve conduction studies were remarkably low to absent. Needle examination showed mild to moderate chronic neuropathic changes in most muscles examined—distal greater than proximal and legs greater than arms. The clinical interpretation was sensorimotor polyneuropathy compatible with the axonal neuropathy seen in Friedreich's ataxia (3).

The patient was confined to a wheelchair at 20 years of age, but attended college and did well in his studies. He had mild trunk and severe limb ataxia, and prominent bilateral pes cavus deformities. He was dysarthric at 20 years and 9 months and he spoke slowly, but he was in his junior year at college with a major in psychology, and was active socially.

Two gait studies were done on this patient—the first at 14 years of age when ataxia became a problem, and the second at 19 years and 10 months, when he lost his ability to walk except in the most protective circumstances (requiring both a walker and an assistant behind to keep him steady enough to move). The two studies portray a progressive course with absence of remissions characteristic in this disease (3).

Film tracings from the left side camera are not remarkable. Film tracings from the front camera showed a variable width of base (Fig. 11.4A—upper portion). The contrast of ankle spread in foot-strike, opposite foot-strike, and foot-strike should be noted, as well as the compensating lateral movements of the arms to provide balance (Fig. 11.4B). It is often said that the ataxic individual has a wider base of support (increased ankle spread). The observations in this laboratory indicate that variability, including both diminished and increased

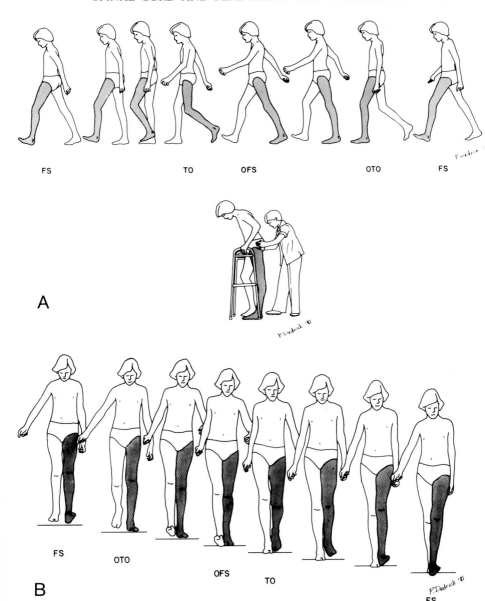

FS   TO OFS   OTO FS

A

FS   OFS   FS
OTO   TO

B

Figure 11.4. (*A* and *B*) Patient P.S., age 14 years: Friedreich's ataxia. (*A*) Tracings (14 years of age) of film from left side camera (upper portion). At 19 years and 10 months of age, patient is unable to stand or walk without the aid of a walker and an assistant (lower portion). (*B*) At 14 years, tracings from front camera film. (See Fig. 11.1 for abbreviations.)

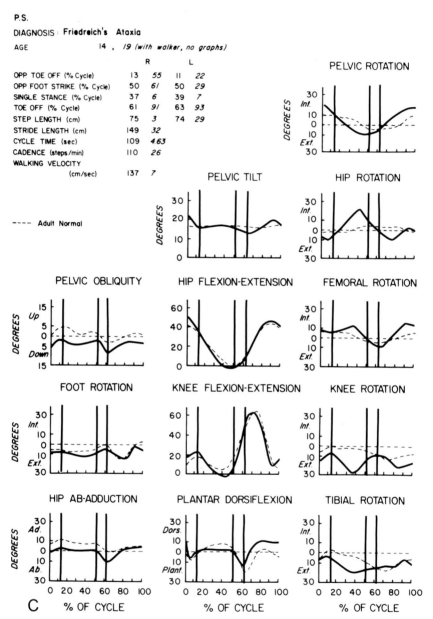

P.S.

DIAGNOSIS : **Friedreich's Ataxia**

AGE   14 , *19 (with walker, no graphs)*

	R	L	
OPP. TOE OFF (% Cycle)	13	*55*	II *22*
OPP FOOT STRIKE (% Cycle)	50	*61*	50 *29*
SINGLE STANCE (% Cycle)	37	*6*	39 *7*
TOE OFF (% Cycle)	61	*91*	63 *93*
STEP LENGTH (cm)	75	*3*	74 *29*
STRIDE LENGTH (cm)	149	*32*		
CYCLE TIME (sec)	109	*463*		
CADENCE (steps/min)	110	*26*		
WALKING VELOCITY (cm/sec)	137	*7*		

- - - - Adult Normal

PELVIC ROTATION

PELVIC TILT

HIP ROTATION

PELVIC OBLIQUITY

HIP FLEXION-EXTENSION

FEMORAL ROTATION

FOOT ROTATION

KNEE FLEXION-EXTENSION

KNEE ROTATION

HIP AB-ADDUCTION

PLANTAR DORSIFLEXION

TIBIAL ROTATION

C   % OF CYCLE   % OF CYCLE   % OF CYCLE

Figure 11.4. (C) Patient P.S. Linear measurements at age 14 and at age 19 years, 10 months. Joint angle rotations, left lower extremity, at age 14 with adult normal values (*dotted line*) for comparison.

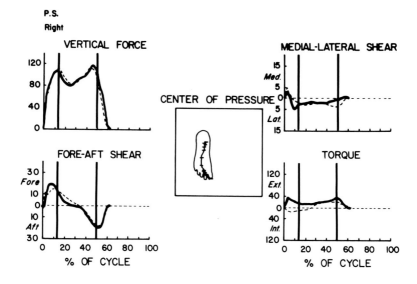

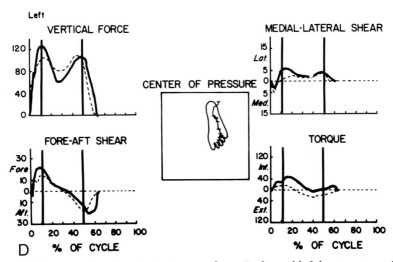

Figure 11.4. (*D*) Patient P.S. at 14 years of age. Right and left lower extremity force plate measurements with adult normal values (*dotted line*) for comparison.

ankle spread, is the hallmark of ataxia. Patients with this disease appear to be constantly staggering, or recovering from an off-balance move. They do not walk with their feet constantly wide apart to avoid a problem. Instead, they react by recovery movements, when difficulties in balance occur. If the ataxia is severe enough, the patient walks near a wall to obtain support when balance is lost.

The marked reduction in patient P.S.'s walking ability is seen in linear measurements at ages 14 and 19 (Fig. 11.4C). Cadence at 14 was 110, but dropped to 26 steps per minute at 19. Walking velocity was 137 cm per second at age 14, dropping to 7 cm per second at age 19. Movement measurements at age 14 show pelvic obliquity with the iliac crest abnormally low in stance phase, with resistive hip abduction, exaggerated internal rotation of the hip, and increased external rotation of the pelvis also in stance phase. The greatest changes of movement occur during single-limb stance, probably due to the ataxia.

The force measurements of the right lower extremity were relatively normal with the exception of torque—internal torque is absent (Fig. 11.4D). The left lower extremity shows exaggerated initial loading, increased forward shear, and loss of external torque in the last half of single-limb stance.

Comparison of joint angle measurements could not be obtained on the second gait study at age 19, since the patient could do little more than stand and shuffle along with maximal support. Tracings from the side camera show attempted ambulation (Fig. 11.3A—lower portion). His height at that time was 6 feet, 3 inches. An electrically powered wheelchair served for household and community ambulation.

References

1. Allan W: Relation of hereditary pattern to clinical severity as illustrated by peroneal atrophy. *Arch Intern Med* 63:1123–1131, 1939.
2. Brooke MH: Diseases of motor neurons. In *A Clinician's View of Neuromuscular Diseases.* Baltimore, Williams & Wilkins, 1977, chap 2, pp 41–43.
3. Drennan JC: Neuromuscular disorders. In Lovell WW, Winter RB: *Pediatric Orthopedics, Vol. I.* Philadelphia, J. B. Lippincott, 1978, Chap 8, pp 312–313.
4. Dyck PJ, Lambert EH: Lower motor and primary sensory neuron diseases with peroneal muscular atrophy. I. Neurologic, genetic and electrophysiologic findings in hereditary polyneuropathies. *Arch Neurol* 18:603–618, 1968.
5. Gardner-Medwin D, Hudgson P, Walton JN: Benign spinal muscular atrophy arising in childhood and adolescence. *J Neurol Sci* 5:121–158, 1967.
6. Kugelberg E, Welander L: Heredofamilial juvenile muscular atrophy simulating muscular dystrophy. *Arch Neurol Psychiatry* 75:500–509, 1956.
7. Levitt RL, Canale ST, Cooke J, et al: The role of foot surgery in progressive neuromuscular disorders in children. *J Bone Joint Surg* 55A:1396–1410, 1973.
8. McKusick VA: The Marfan syndrome. In *Heritable Disorders of Connective Tissue.* St. Louis, C. V. Mosby, 1972, chap 3, pp 61–223.

CHAPTER 12

Chronic Arthritis

INTRODUCTION

Many diseases can produce arthritis in children—for example, cases of nonspecific synovitis, Legg-Calvé-Perthes disease, and foreign body synovitis as presented in Chapter 6. Other disease processes such as septic arthritis, acute rheumatic fever, leukemia, systemic lupus erythematosus, polyarthritis with regional enteritis, polyarteritis nodosa and dermatomyositis must be included in the differential diagnosis. Synovial hemangioma can produce bouts of recurring synovitis secondary to intra-articular bleeds.

Chronic arthritis in children is most frequently due to rheumatoid arthritis or hemophilia. The subject of this chapter will be the gait abnormalities found in these two disease entities.

There are three clinical forms of juvenile rheumatoid arthritis: monoarticular or pauciarticular arthritis, polyarthritis, and polyarthritis with an acute febrile onset. Pauciarticular arthritis involves more than one, but less than four joints. Polyarthritis (Still's disease) involves four or more joints for a minimal duration of 3 months. If fewer joints are affected, synovial biopsy must show changes compatible with the diagnosis of rheumatoid arthritis (2).

Children with the monoarticular or pauciarticular form ordinarily do not have fever, rash, or enlargement of the spleen or liver. The erythrocyte sedimentation rate may be elevated, but often is not, and the serum latex fixation test is usually negative. Iridocyclitis is more common in this variety, and ophthalmological examination must be included (1, 2). Severe and permanent vision impairment can result without proper treatment.

In polyarthritis, there is a higher incidence of cervical spine involvement with relatively higher titers for the rheumatoid factor and antinuclear antibodies. The prognosis is less favorable in this form than in monoarticular or pauciarticular arthritis.

The image that comes to mind when the subject of juvenile rheumatoid arthritis is mentioned is the small child with multiple thickened joints, muscle wasting, and joint contractures. Although this is the characteristic presentation of a severely involved juvenile arthritic (11), many children with this disease make complete recovery. As compared with adults who have rheumatoid arthritis, juvenile rheumatoid arthritics have a more favorable prognosis. Five years after onset, half of the patients followed by Ansell and Bywaters (1) had no residual lesions of the joints, and two-thirds were clinically inactive with a sedimentation rate of less than 20 mm per hour.

The joint changes in chronic juvenile rheumatoid arthritis depend upon the intensity of the process, duration of involvement, age of the child, and the joints involved. Medical management includes aspirin, rest, physical therapy, and splinting of the joints to avoid contractures. Gold may be added if aspirin does not control the inflammation. Corticosteroids are used in treating iridocyclitis. Otherwise, long-term steroid administration should be avoided because of side effects such as: increased susceptibility to infection, occurrence of vertebral fractures, moon facies, and obesity. Surgical synovectomy may help to reduce joint pain and swelling when medical treatment measures have failed (5), but the primary risk with synovectomy is loss of motion. Two significant developments in orthopaedic surgery in the last decade may reduce the risk of motion loss as a complication of synovectomy. The synovia can be removed through an arthroscope, and there is much less postoperative pain and disability (8). Continuous passive motion begun immediately after surgery speeds recovery of function and maintains the motion range achieved during surgery (10). No long-term results have been reported as yet, using either of these treatment modalities for juvenile rheumatoid arthritis. However, any surgeon contemplating arthrotomy and synovectomy in this disease should consider including continuous passive motion in the postoperative management. Whether synovectomy can be accomplished in a satisfactory manner through an arthroscope is a question still to be resolved (7).

Gait abnormalities in juvenile rheumatoid arthritis can include limping, reduction in step length, cadence and velocity, and restricted joint motion. Some children are unable to walk during acute episodes, but most can walk with impairment.

JUVENILE RHEUMATOID ARTHRITIS

Patient M.V. was well until the age of 7, when she began to complain of some discomfort in her hands and feet. Daily temperature elevations were noted; her appetite decreased, and she began to lose weight. She was hospitalized for diagnostic studies which were as follows: hemoglobin, 9.3 g; white blood count, 16,900; differential blood count: 65 polymorphonuclear leukocytes, 32 lymphocytes, 3 eosinophils; initial sedimentation rate, 29; latex fixation test negative; ASTO titer less than 166 Todd units; febrile agglutinins normal; urinalysis, 5–7 white blood cells. Bone marrow aspiration showed moderate thrombocytosis and mild normocytic normochromic anemia.

At that time, range of motion of the extremities had not decreased significantly, but palpation of the wrists and fingers disclosed some tenderness. Following initial hospitalization, the patient was placed on aspirin, but began to experience pain in multiple joints and developed stiffness in her knees, hips and hands. Knee joint fluid had a turbid appearance, and the mucin clot was poor. White blood cells were 4293 per cu mm, and the differential blood count showed 70% polymorphonuclear leukocytes. A diagnosis of juvenile rheumatoid arthritis was established.

The treatment program included daily aspirin to therapeutic levels, weekly injections of gold (Myochrysine), and steroids were given for a short time. A physical therapy program was started early, but the patient lived some distance away from the hospital and did not maintain a regular program. Medications were taken faithfully.

Physical examination revealed a small child who appeared chronically ill. Motion was significantly restricted in both hips.

	Right	Left
Hips:		
Flexion	90	80
Extension	−30	−25
Abduction	45	−20
Knee:		
Flexion	120	120
Extension	0	0
Ankle dorsiflexion	20	20

Film tracings from the side camera showed joint thickening about the knees, quadriceps atrophy, restricted right and left step length (Fig. 12.1A). Film tracings from the front camera showed right and left antalgic hip gait (gluteus medius lurch) (Fig. 12.1B).

Walking velocity and cadence were slow, and step lengths were asymmetrical (Fig. 12.1C). The right step length was 32 cm, and the left, 22 cm. Duration of single stance was 33 for each lower extremity. The joint angle rotations of the left lower extremity showed marked abnormalities (Fig. 12.1C). The hip remained flexed throughout the cycle. There was increased knee flexion in stance phase, as well as increased pelvic obliquity and hip abduction throughout the cycle. Pelvic rotation showed a pattern of exaggerated external rotation, and the hip showed increased internal rotation throughout the cycle. The most striking abnormalities of movement were: limited hip motion with the hip maintained in flexion, pelvic obliquity with the left pelvic crest low, and excessive left hip abduction throughout the cycle.

The slow cadence and velocity (78 steps per minute and 15 cm per second) and the restricted motion in the left hip are entirely consistent

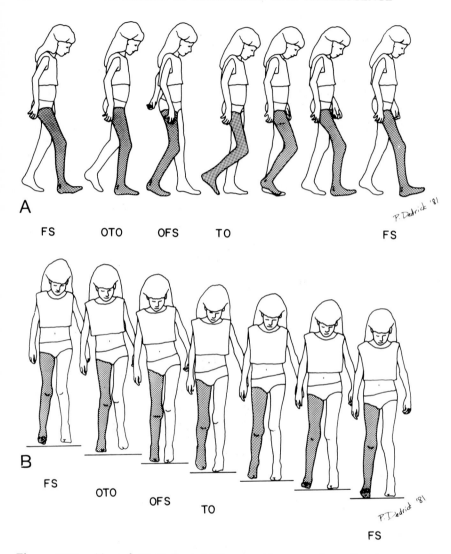

Figure 12.1. (*A* and *B*) Patient M.V., age 10 years: Juvenile rheumatoid arthritis. Tracings of film from right side (*A*) and front (*B*) camera. (FS = foot-strike, OTO = opposite toe-off, OFS = opposite foot-strike, and TO = toe-off.)

with the history and physical findings. X-rays of the hips revealed advanced degenerative changes which will necessitate total hip arthroplasties in the future (Fig. 12.1*D*).

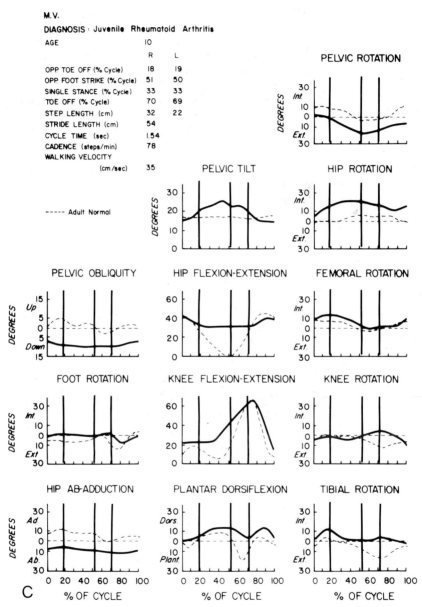

Figure 12.1. (C) Patient M.V. Linear measurements and joint angle rotations, right lower extremity. Joint angle rotations are compared with values for normal adult.

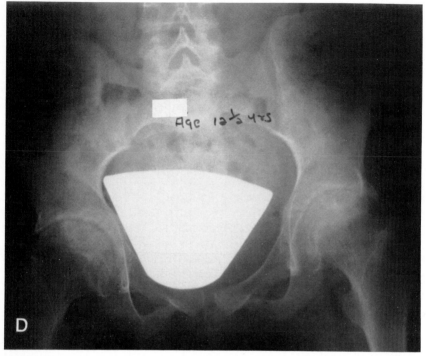

Figure 12.1. (*D*) Patient M.V. at 12½ years of age. AP pelvic x-ray shows bilateral marked joint narrowing and lytic lesions in the femoral heads.

HEMOPHILIA

Estimates of the incidence of hemophilia vary from 1 in 10,000 to 1 in 100,000. Development of effective concentrates for classic hemophilia A and hemophilia B (Christmas disease) has resulted in a more favorable prognosis for bleeding control. In spite of available treatment methods, neither prompt treatment nor joint aspirations can completely prevent arthritis. Prophylactic therapy can impede changes in the joints, but this carries the risk of producing antibodies which inhibit the effectiveness of the factor concentrates. Joint changes in hemophiliac arthropathy vary in severity. There are three stages: Stage I, simple arthrosis, with synovial thickening, excessive deposits of hemosiderin in the synovium, and fibrosis; Stage II, pan-arthritis—progressive cartilage erosion and bone-to-bone adhesions (muscle contractures and limited motion are common in this stage); and Stage III, some regression and organization with proliferation of fibrous connective tissue, subchondral bone cysts, and restricted motion. Knee joint changes in Stage III include narrowing of the joint space, punched-out areas over joint surfaces, deepening and widening of the intercondylar notch, bone atrophy, synovial thickening and pigmentation (6, 12). The hip joint is particularly vulnerable because avascular necrosis often occurs, producing deformation of the femoral head and limb length inequality.

An experimental study on dogs by Convery and others (4) may explain the mechanism of cartilage degeneration in hemophilia. The knee joints of skeletally mature mongrel dogs were injected 5 times weekly with heparinized autologous blood in one knee for periods from 4 to 16 weeks. The opposite knee joint was injected with heparinized saline to act as a control. The animals were sacrificed at 4, 8, 12 and 16 weeks, and the joint surfaces were subjected to biochemical analyses and bioengineering measurements of the cartilage surfaces. A significant decrease in the glycosaminoglycans, expressed as hexosamine, was progressively evident throughout the study. A corresponding decrease in shear resistance in the cartilage was positively correlated with the reduction in hexosamine. The conclusion was that repeated bleeds into the joint can alter the glycosaminoglycan structure of the cartilage, leading to decreased resistance to shear and progressive cartilage damage. The other changes in the joint were brown staining of the synovium and articular cartilage. In the 12- and 16-week specimens, variable thickening of the fibrous capsule and synovial hypertrophy were noted. In some specimens, the synovium encroached across the cartilage margin.

Gait abnormalities in hemophilia include limping, restricted motion, and alterations in velocity and cadence. When pain is not a factor, there may be little or no limp, and motion impairment may be the only visual clue to existence of joint damage. A short-limb gait may be recognized by excessive drop of the ipsilateral pelvis crest or may, of course, be more easily detected when a shoe elevation is worn.

As is the case in juvenile rheumatoid arthritis, advocates of synovectomy in treating hemophiliac arthropathy are chiefly orthopaedic surgeons (5). The problem of timing for this procedure is crucial. When synovectomy is performed too early, it serves no purpose, since medical management is usually sufficient. Synovectomy after the joint has been destroyed is equally ineffective. Current management includes aggressive medical control of bleeding, an active physical therapy program to maintain muscle strength and avoid contractures, synovectomy of painful boggy joints with recurrent hemorrhages refractory to medical management (5, 9), and total joint arthroplasty for patients disabled by complete joint destruction.

Hemophiliac Arthropathy

Patient S.V. is the younger of two brothers with severe classic hemophilia (Factor VIII deficiency). The diagnosis was made at age 2 months, and he remained under continuous care of the hemophilia management team. The left hip was the site of one of the earliest bleeds, and left hip symptoms continued intermittently after the initial episode. The patient was placed on a home treatment program with regular follow-up. While there were bleeds into multiple joints, the right ankle, left hip, and right elbow were most frequently involved. X-rays revealed destruction of the capital femoral epiphysis and a gradual trochanteric overgrowth. Shoe elevation was required for progressive shortening of the left lower extremity. At the age of 11, the patient underwent right distal femoral epiphyseodesis to correct the leg length inequality. When he was 15, excision of the right radial head relieved chronic symptoms in the right elbow.

A gait study was done when the patient was 16 years of age. His height was 5 feet, 7 inches, and he required a ½-inch block under the left foot to level his pelvis. A pelvic x-ray revealed trochanteric overgrowth and partial destruction of the femoral head (Fig. 12.2A).

Examination revealed the following:

	Right	Left
Hip motion:		
Flexion	95	90
Extension	−5	−5
Abduction	25	10
Adduction	20	20
Internal rotation	45	45
External rotation	30	0
Knee flexion	140	145
Knee extension	0	−5
Ankle dorsiflexion	10	5

The patient experienced some pain in the right ankle and could not raise his heel from the floor with his entire weight on the right lower extremity. The medical treatment plan in operation at the time of the study was home use of Factor VIII only when bleeds occurred.

Film tracings from the left side camera showed ankle equinus during single-limb support and diminished left hip extension in stance phase (Fig. 12.2B). Film tracings from the front camera showed shoulder sway and drop of the contralateral pelvic crest during stance phase (gluteus medius lurch) (Fig. 12.2C). Walking velocity, cadence and stride length were 131, 122, and 128 cm, respectively, compared with adult normal values of 126, 111, and 135 cm (Fig. 12.2D). Anterior pelvic tilt was exaggerated, and the hip remained flexed throughout the cycle. Exaggerated knee flexion and ankle equinus were present during single-limb stance. The pelvis was externally rotated throughout the cycle, with marked internal rotation of the hip. Pelvic obliquity

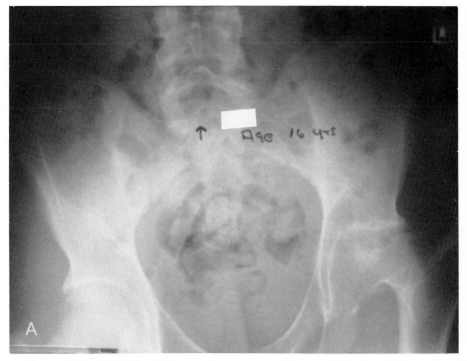

Figure 12.2. (A) Patient S.V., age 16 years: classic hemophilia. Partial destruction of left femoral head with marked trochanteric overgrowth.

was exaggerated, with the left pelvic crest high throughout the single-limb stance (Fig. 12.2D).

In summary, motion abnormalities were evident at hip, knee and ankle. The hip remained flexed and internally rotated. The pelvis remained in external rotation, in an attitude of increased anterior pelvic tilt. Knee flexion and ankle plantar flexion were magnified during stance phase.

Force plate measurements of the right lower extremity showed exaggerated loading and increased second peak vertical force (Fig. 12.2E). Lateral shear increased slightly—a normal center of pressure progression pattern. Initial loading and lateral shear were exaggerated in the left lower extremity, and diminished second peak vertical force and an equinovalgus pattern of center of pressure progression were noted.

In spite of these gait abnormalities, walking velocity indicated a well-compensated gait, and pain was not sufficient to warrant orthopaedic intervention. The left hip joint has been seriously compromised,

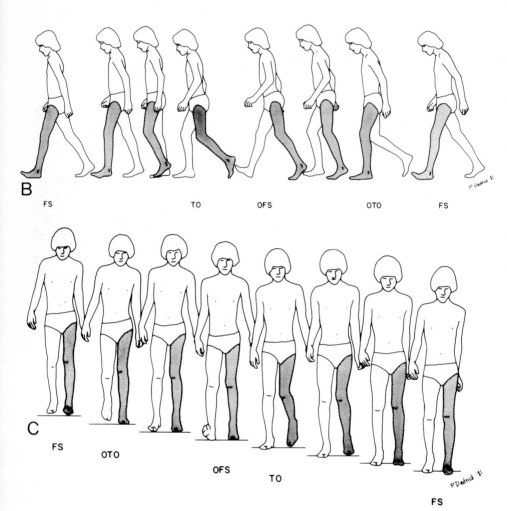

B

FS   TO   OFS   OTO   FS

C

FS

     OTO

                  OFS

                        TO

                                       FS

Figure 12.2.   (*B* and *C*) Patient S.V. Tracings from left (*B*) and front (*C*) camera film. (See Fig. 12.1 for abbreviations.)

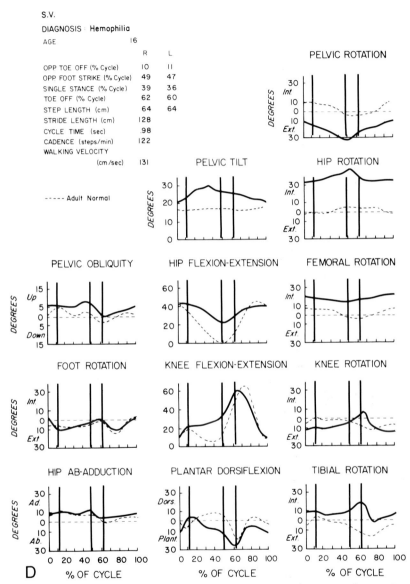

Figure 12.2. (*D*) Patient S.V. Linear measurements and joint angle rotations, left lower extremity. Joint angle rotations are compared with normal adult values.

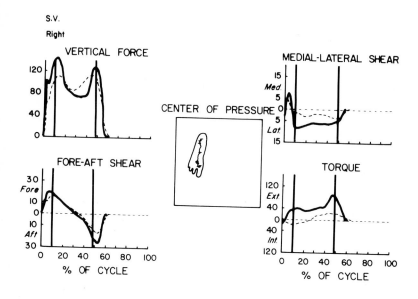

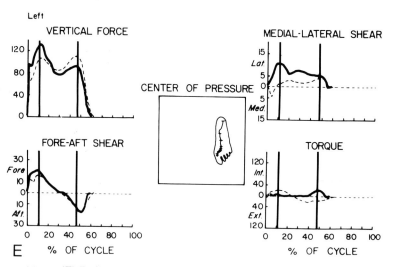

Figure 12.2.   (E) Patient S.V. Force plate measurements, right and left lower extremities, compared to adult normal values.

however, and total hip arthroplasty will be done when pain requires it. This procedure will be delayed as long as possible to reduce the chances of loosening. The loosening rate for total hip arthroplasties in younger individuals is high (3).

References

1. Ansell BM, Bywaters EGL: Rheumatoid arthritis (Still's disease). *Pediatr Clin North Am* 10:921–939, 1963.
2. Bianco AJ: Juvenile rheumatoid arthritis and ankylosing spondylitis. In Lovell WW, Winter RB: *Pediatric Orthopedics, Vol. I.* Philadelphia, W. B. Lippincott, 1978, pp 449–474.
3. Chandler HP, McCarthy JC, Reineck FT, et al: Total hip replacement in patients younger than 30 years of age—a five-year follow-up. *J Bone Joint Surg* 63A:1426–1434, 1981.
4. Convery FR, Woo SLY, Akeson WH, et al: Experimental hemarthrosis in the knee of the mature canine. *Arthritis Rheum* 19:59–67, 1976.
5. Eyring EJ, Lingert A, Bass J: Synovectomy in juvenile rheumatoid arthritis. Indications and short-term results. *J Bone Joint Surg* 63:638, 1971.
6. Lofthouse RN: Bone changes in hemophilia. *J Bone Joint Surg* 39B:794, 1957.
7. Matsui N, Moriya H, Kitahara H: The use in arthroscopy for follow-up in knee joint surgery. *Orthop Clin North Am* 10:697–708, 1976.
8. O'Connor RL: The synovium. In *Arthroscopy.* Philadelphia, J. B. Lippincott, 1977, Chap 4, pp 36–37.
9. Pietrogrande VD, Dioguardi N, Mannucci PM: Short-term evaluation of synovectomy in hemophilia. *Br Med J* 2:378–381, 1972.
10. Salter RB, Simmonds DF, Malcolm BW, et al: The biological effect of continuous passive motion on the healing of full-thickness defects in articular cartilage. *J Bone Joint Surg* 62A:1232–1251, 1980.
11. Still GF: On a form of chronic joint disease in children. *Med Chir Trans* 80:45, 1897.
12. Trueta J: Haemophilia. In *Studies of the Development and Decay of the Human Frame.* Philadelphia, W. B. Saunders, 1968, Chap 29, pp 238–253.

Index